The
Big Book of
Clinical Research Unraveled

The Big Book of Clinical Research Unraveled

Keys for the Puzzles Based on Clinical Research Topics

Crosswords I Jumbled Words I Word Search I Odd-One-Out I Process Flows

Sanjay Gupta

CR Books

First published in India by
CR Books Pvt. Ltd.
503, NDM-2, Netaji Subhash Place, Pitampura, Delhi-110034
Tel: +91-11-45121445 Fax : +91-11-45121435
E-mail : info@crbooks.net, info@crbooks.us
Web : www.crbooks.net

First Edition : January 2012

The author and publisher have made a conscientious effort to ensure that the information contained in this book is accurate and in accordance with the accepted standards at the time of publication. However, in this rapidly changing world guidelines and practices are subject to change without prior notification, therefore readers are advised to confirm these as and when needed.

Printed and bound by Elite Printer
eliteprinter@yahoo.in

ISBN 81-922277-1-5

Contents

Preface

The Big Book of Clinical Research was published in January 2011 with the aim to serve as a workbook for fun learning through crosswords, jumbled words, word search, odd-one-out and process flows based on clinical research topics. The book has received wide acclamation and a need was felt to have the solutions in order to evaluate as well as to enhance the competency level of clinical research professionals.

The present book contains the solutions of crosswords, jumbled words, word search, odd-one-out and process flows featured in the Big Book of Clinical Research. I hope the book would be helpful in evaluating the competency level of people for a particular job level.

12th January 2012

Sanjay Gupta

1

Keys for Crosswords

This section contains solution of 150 crossword puzzles. For the ease of readers abbreviations have been elaborated at the bottom of the solutions.

Crossword # 1

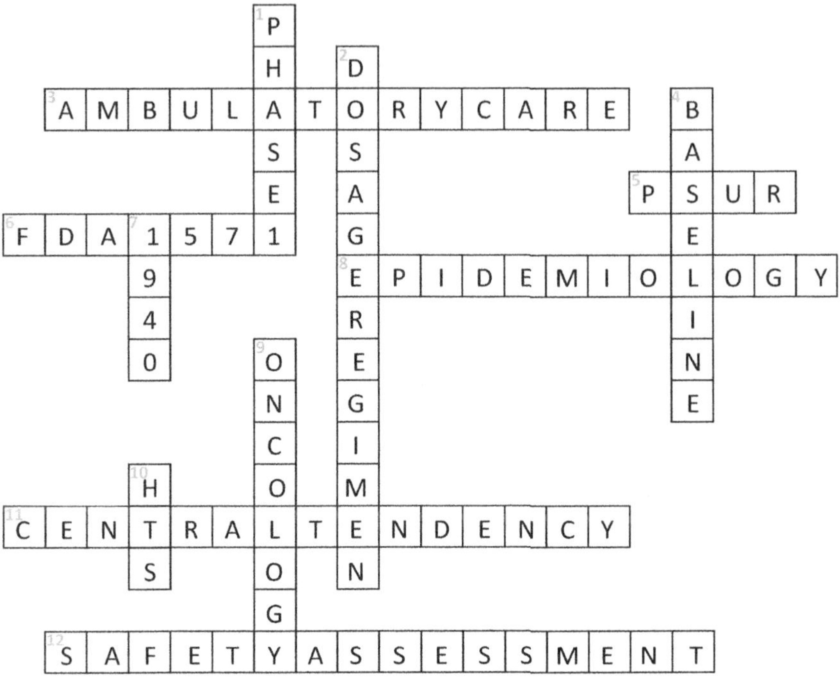

Across

3. AMBULATORY CARE
5. PSUR
6. FDA1571
8. EPIDEMIOLOGY
11. CENTRAL TENDENCY
12. SAFETY ASSESSMENT

Down

1. PHASE 1
2. DOSAGE REGIMEN
4. BASELINE
7. 1940
9. ONCOLOGY
10. HTS

PSUR: Periodic Safety Update Report; **HTS**: High Throughput Screening

Crossword # 2

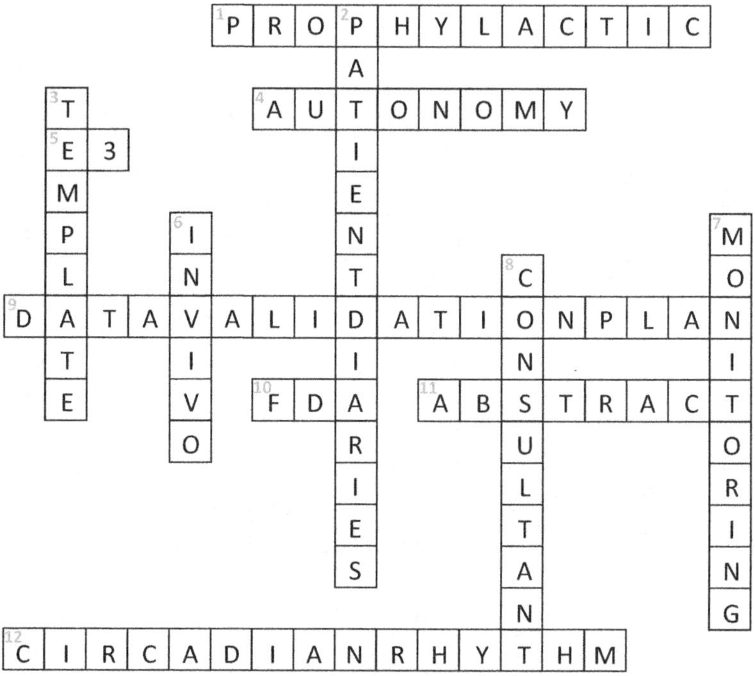

Across

1. PROPHYLACTIC
4. AUTONOMY
5. E3
9. DATA VALIDATION PLAN
10. FDA
11. ABSTRACT
12. CIRCADIAN RHYTHM

Down

2. PATIENT DIARIES
3. TEMPLATE
6. INVIVO
7. MONITORING
8. CONSULTANT

Crossword # 3

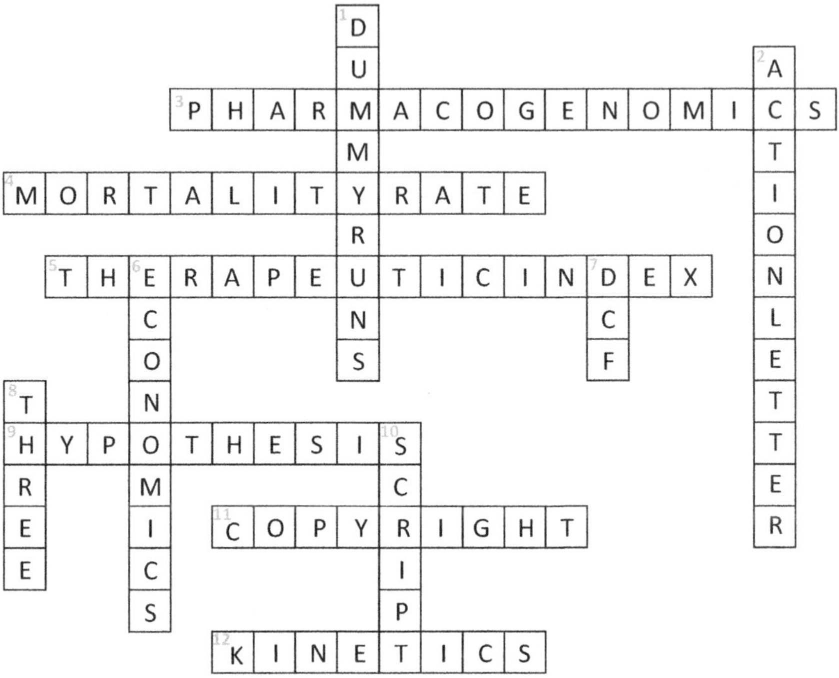

Across

3. PHARMACOGENOMICS
4. MORTALITY RATE
5. THERAPEUTIC INDEX
9. HYPOTHESIS
11. COPYRIGHT
12. KINETICS

Down

1. DUMMY RUNS
2. ACTION LETTER
6. ECONOMICS
7. DCF
8. THREE
10. SCRIPT

DCF: Data Clarification Form

Crossword # 4

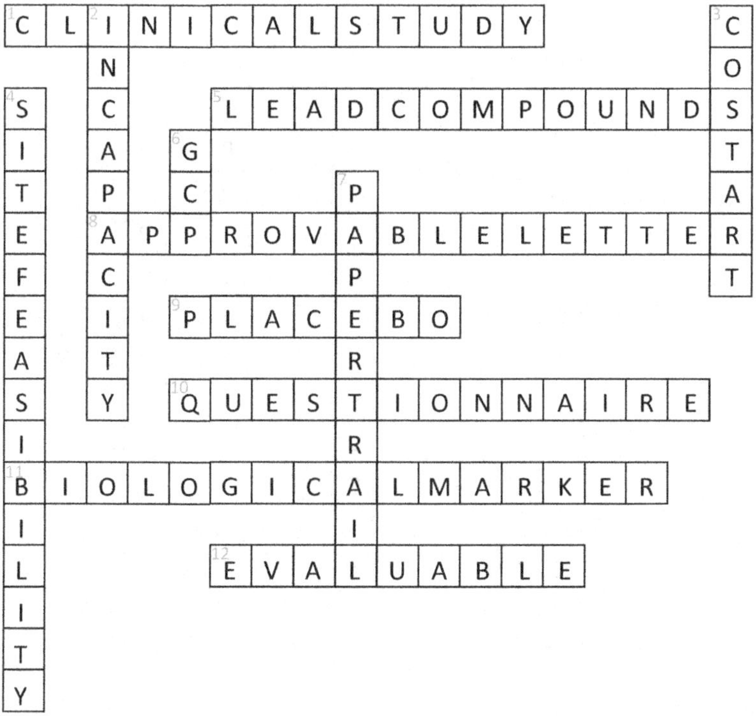

Across

1. CLINICAL STUDY
5. LEAD COMPOUNDS
8. APPROVABLE LETTER
9. PLACEBO
10. QUESTIONNAIRE
11. BIOLOGICAL MARKER
12. EVALUABLE

Down

2. INCAPACITY
3. COSTART
4. SITE FEASIBILITY
6. GCP
7. PAPER TRAIL

GCP: Good Clinical Practice

Crossword # 5

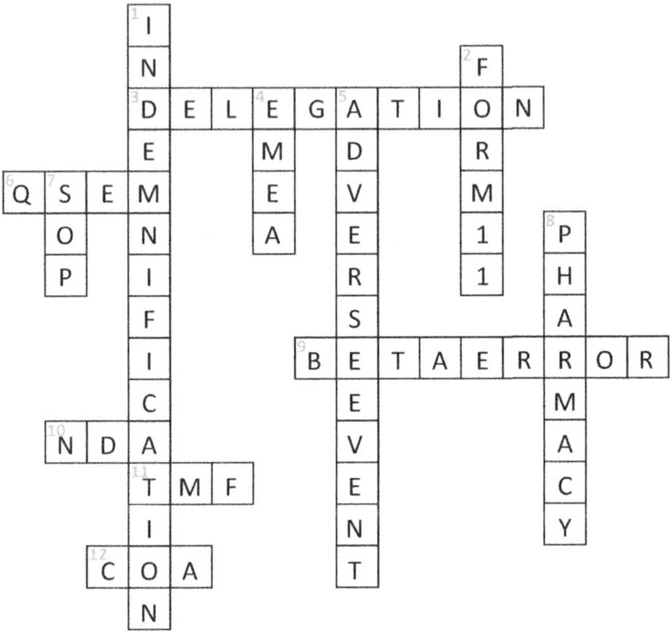

Across

3. DELEGATION
6. QSEM
9. BETA ERROR
10. NDA
11. TMF
12. COA

Down

1. INDEMNIFICATION
2. FORM 11
4. EMEA
5. ADVERSE EVENT
7. SOP
8. PHARMACY

QSEM: Quality, Safety, Efficacy, Multidisciplinary ; **NDA**: Non Disclosure Agreement; **TMF**: Trial Master File; **COA**: Certificate of Analysis; **EMEA**: European Agency for the Evaluation of Medicinal Products; **SOP**: Standard Operating Procedure

Crossword # 6

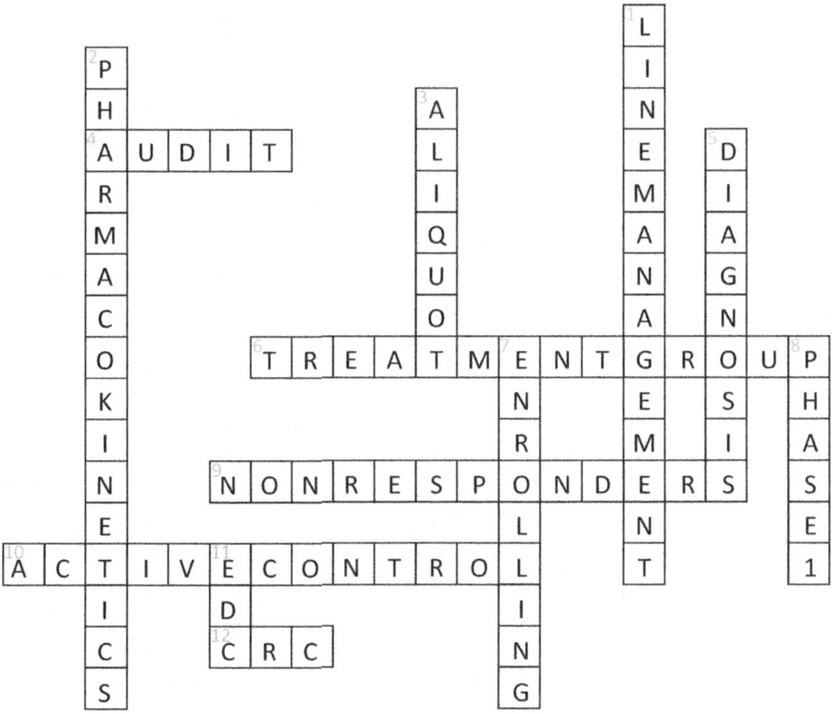

Across

4. AUDIT
6. TREATMENT GROUP
9. NON RESPONDERS
10. ACTIVE CONTROL
12. CRC

Down

1. LINE MANAGEMENT
2. PHARMACOKINETICS
3. ALIQUOT
5. DIAGNOSIS
7. ENROLLING
8. PHASE 1
11. EDC

CRC: Clinical Research Coordinator; **EDC**: Electronic Data Capture

Crossword # 7

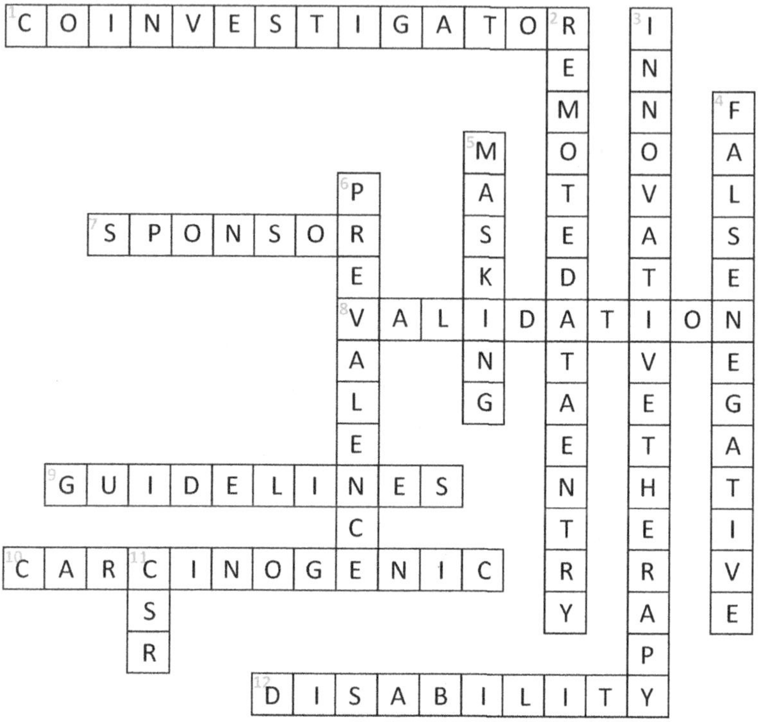

Across

1. COINVESTIGATOR
7. SPONSOR
8. VALIDATION
9. GUIDELINES
10. CARCINOGENIC
12. DISABILITY

Down

2. REMOTE DATA ENTRY
3. INNOVATIVE THERAPY
4. FALSE NEGATIVE
5. MASKING
6. PREVALENCE
11. CSR

CSR: Clinical Study Report

Crossword # 8

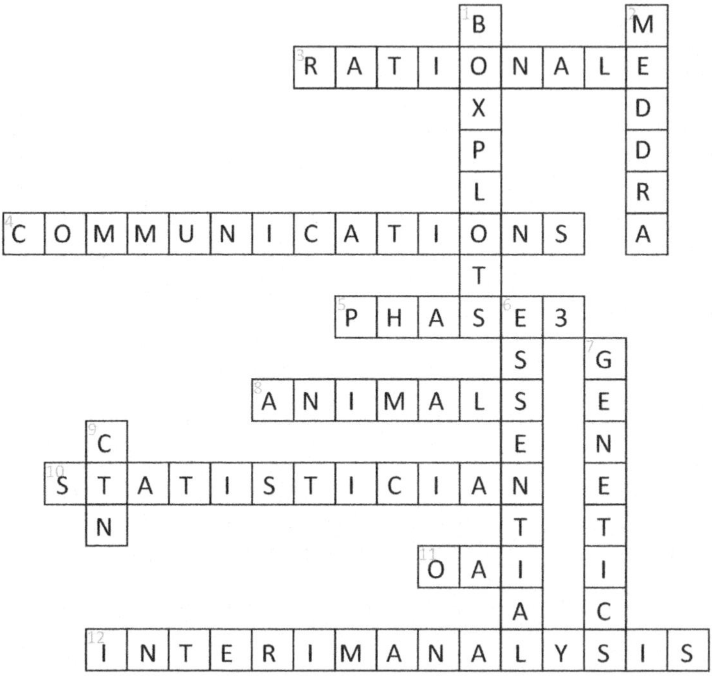

Across

3. RATIONALE
4. COMMUNICATIONS
5. PHASE 3
8. ANIMALS
10. STATISTICIAN
11. OAI
12. INTERIM ANALYSIS

Down

1. BOXPLOTS
2. MedDRA
6. ESSENTIAL
7. GENETICS
9. CTN

OAI: Official Action Indicated; **MedDRA**: Medical Dictionary for Regulatory Activities

Crossword # 9

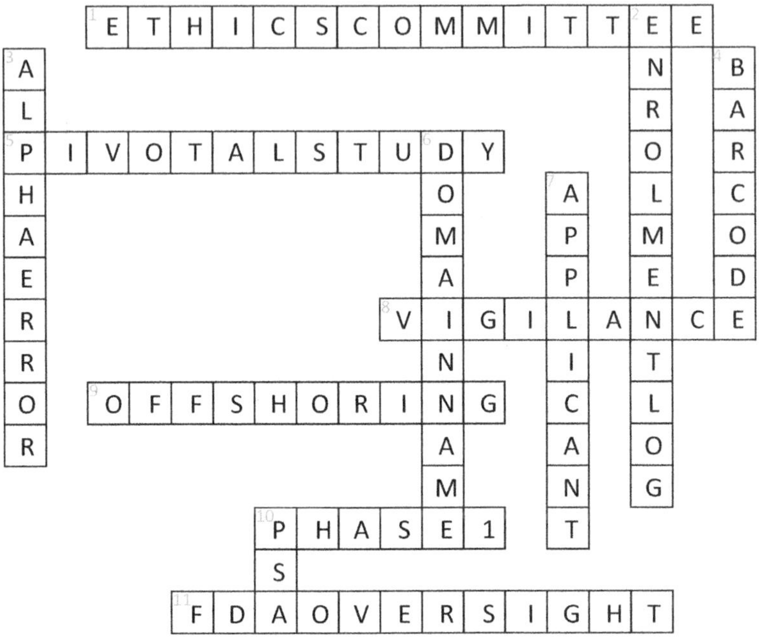

Across

1. ETHICS COMMITTEE
5. PIVOTAL STUDY
8. VIGILANCE
9. OFF SHORING
10. PHASE 1
11. FDA OVERSIGHT

Down

2. ENROLMENT LOG
3. ALPHA ERROR
4. BARCODE
6. DOMAIN NAME
7. APPLICANT
10. PSA

PSA: Professional Services Agreement

Crossword # 10

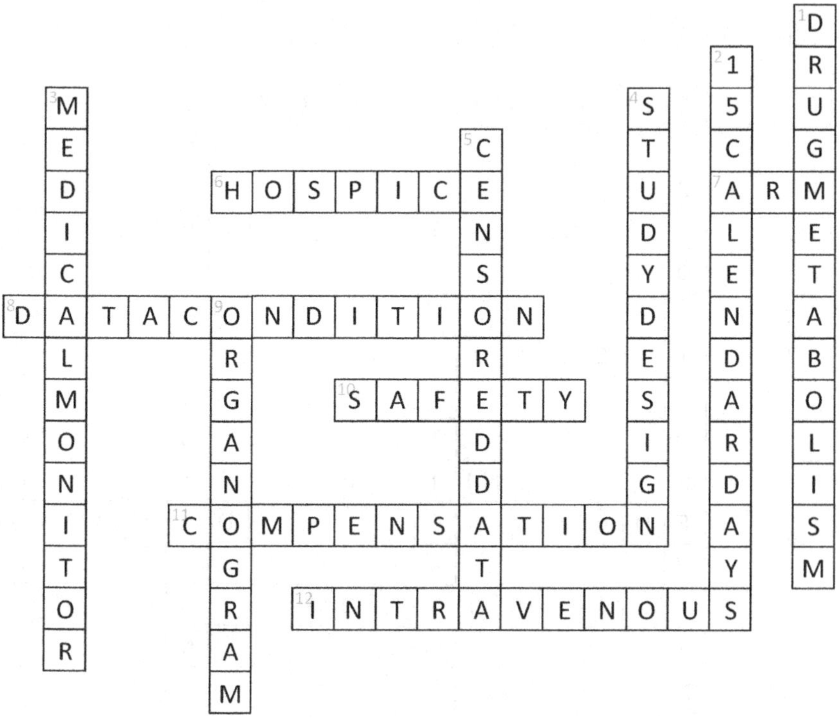

Across

6. HOSPICE
7. ARM
8. DATA CONDITION
10. SAFETY
11. COMPENSATION
12. INTRAVENOUS

Down

1. DRUG METABOLISM
2. 15 CALENDAR DAYS
3. MEDICAL MONITOR
4. STUDY DESIGN
5. CENSORED DATA
9. ORGANOGRAM

Crossword # 11

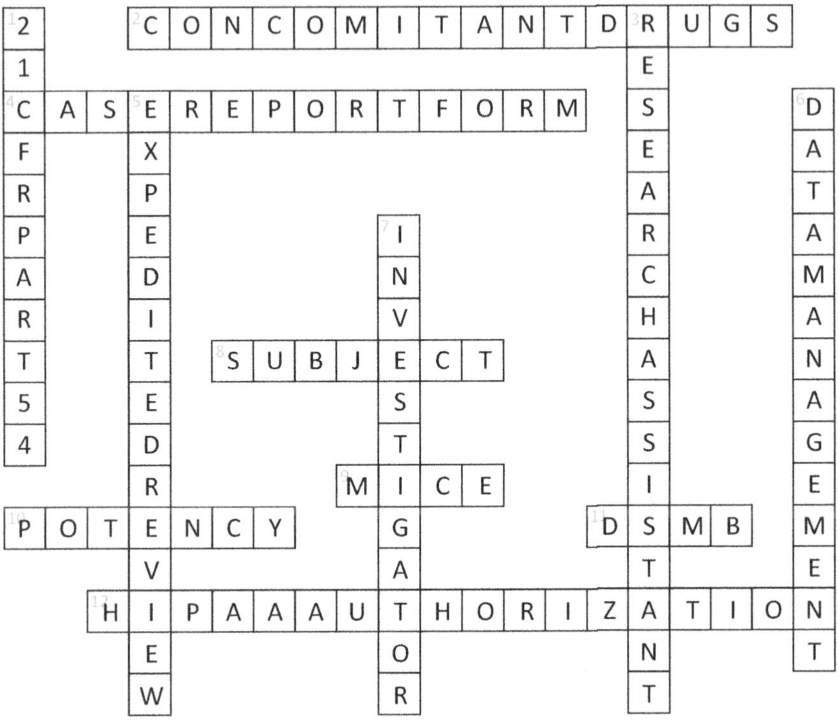

Across

2. CONCOMITANT DRUGS
4. CASE REPORT FORM
8. SUBJECT
9. MICE
10. POTENCY
11. DSMB
12. HIPAA AUTHORIZATION

Down

1. 21 CFR PART 54
3. RESEARCH ASSISTANT
5. EXPEDITED REVIEW
6. DATA MANAGEMENT
7. INVESTIGATOR

DSMB: Data Safety Monitoring Board; **HIPAA**: Health Insurance Portability and Accountability Act

Crossword # 12

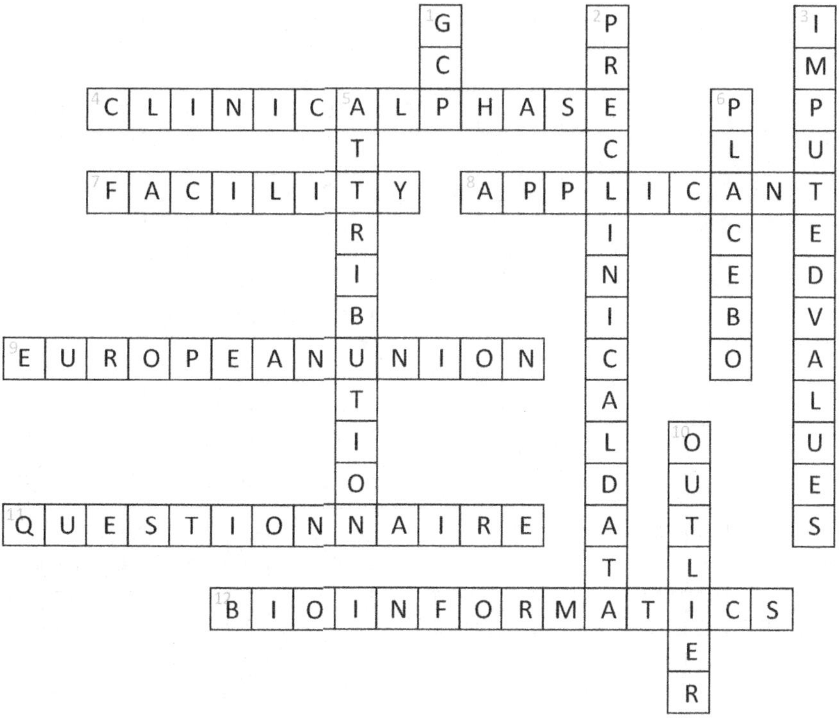

Across

4. CLINICAL PHASE
7. FACILITY
8. APPLICANT
9. EUROPEAN UNION
11. QUESTIONNAIRE
12. BIOINFORMATICS

Down

1. GCP
2. PRE CLINICAL DATA
3. IMPUTED VALUES
5. ATTRIBUTION
6. PLACEBO
10. OUTLIER

GCP: Good Clinical Practice

Crossword # 13

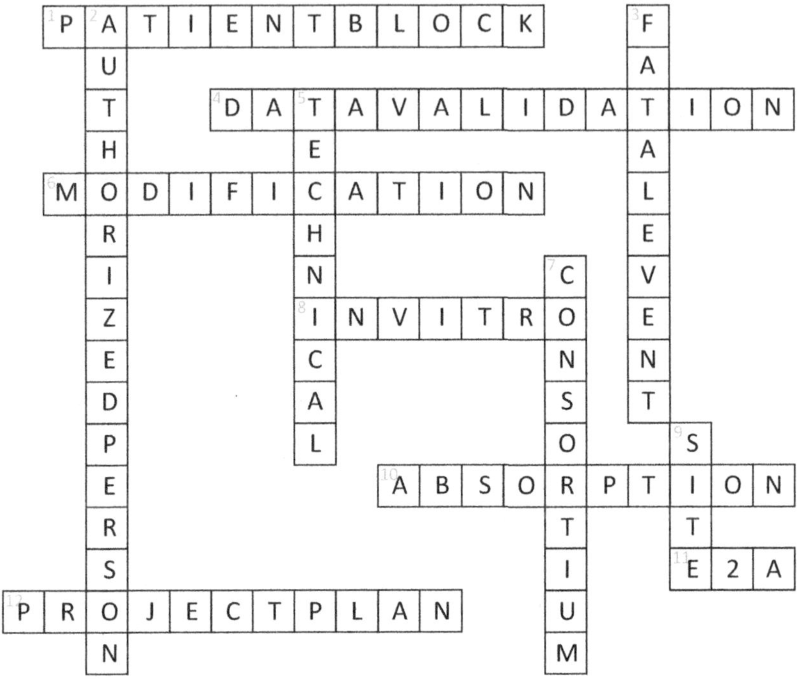

Across

1. PATIENT BLOCK
4. DATA VALIDATION
6. MODIFICATION
8. IN VITRO
10. ABSORPTION
11. E2A
12. PROJECT PLAN

Down

2. AUTHORIZED PERSON
3. FATAL EVENT
5. TECHNICAL
7. CONSORTIUM
9. SITE

Crossword # 14

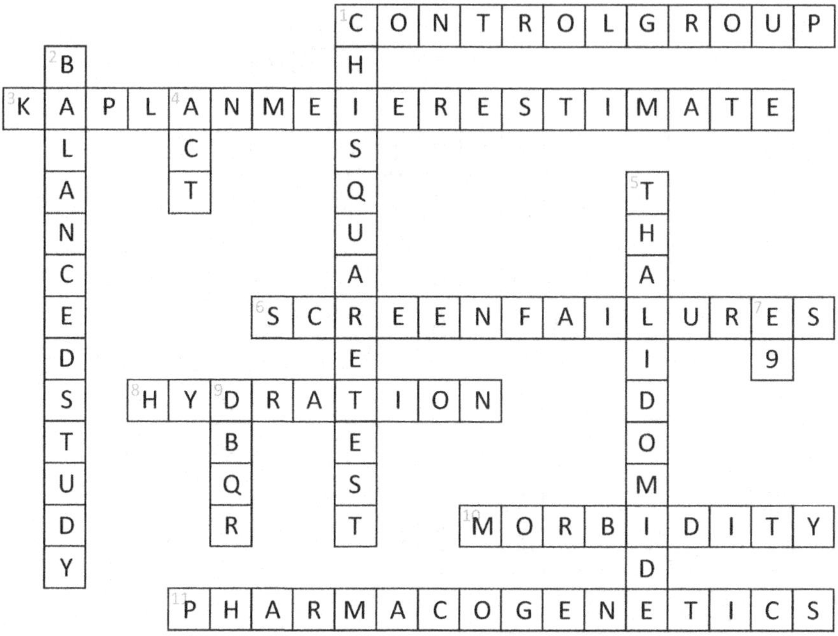

Across

1. CONTROL GROUP
3. KAPLAN MEIER ESTIMATE
6. SCREEN FAILURES
8. HYDRATION
10. MORBIDITY
11. PHARMACOGENETICS

Down

1. CHI SQUARE TEST
2. BALANCED STUDY
4. ACT
5. THALIDOMIDE
7. E9
9. DBQR

DBQR: Database Quality Review

Crossword # 15

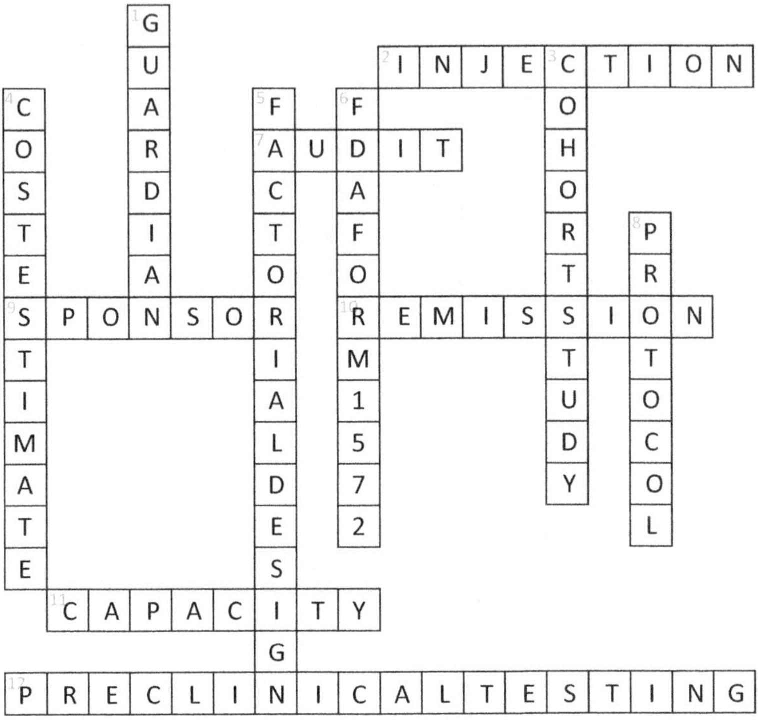

Across

2. INJECTION
7. AUDIT
9. SPONSOR
10. REMISSION
11. CAPACITY
12. PRE CLINICAL TESTING

Down

1. GUARDIAN
3. COHORT STUDY
4. COST ESTIMATE
5. FACTORIAL DESIGN
6. FDA FORM 1572
8. PROTOCOL

FDA: Food and Drug Administration

Crossword # 16

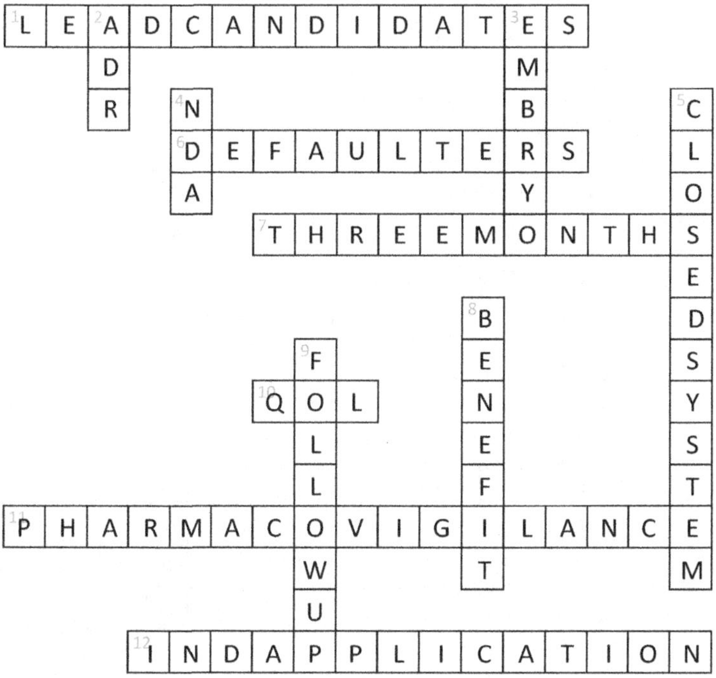

Across

1. LEAD CANDIDATES
6. DEFAULTERS
7. THREE MONTHS
10. QOL
11. PHARMACOVIGILANCE
12. IND APPLICATION

Down

2. ADR
3. EMBRYO
4. NDA
5. CLOSED SYSTEM
8. BENEFIT
9. FOLLOW UP

QOL: Quality of Life; **ADR**: Adverse Drug Reaction; **NDA**: New Drug Application

Crossword # 17

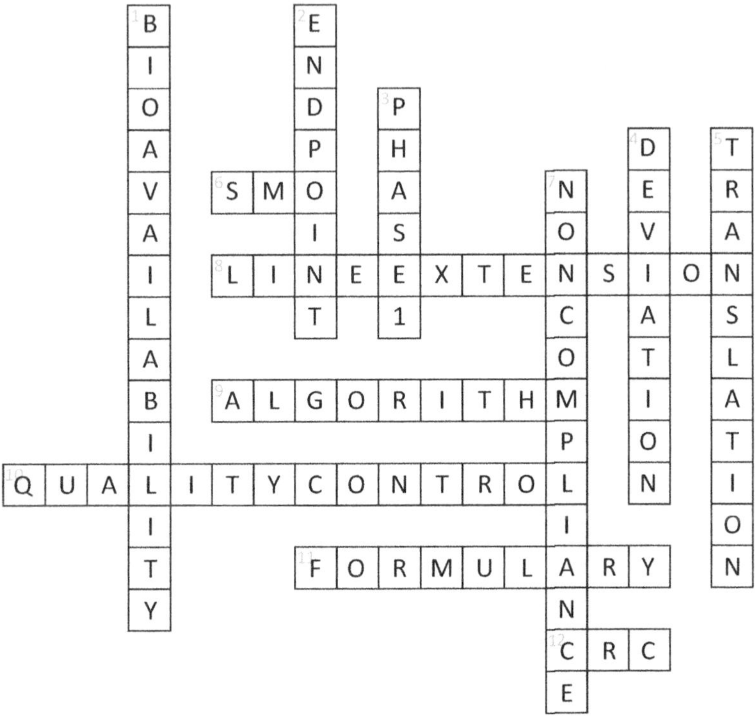

Across

6. SMO
8. LINE EXTENSION
9. ALGORITHM
10. QUALITY CONTROL
11. FORMULARY
12. CRC

Down

1. BIOAVAILABILITY
2. ENDPOINT
3. PHASE 1
4. DEVIATION
5. TRANSLATION
7. NON COMPLIANCE

SMO: Site Management Organization; **CRC**: Clinical Research Coordinator

Crossword # 18

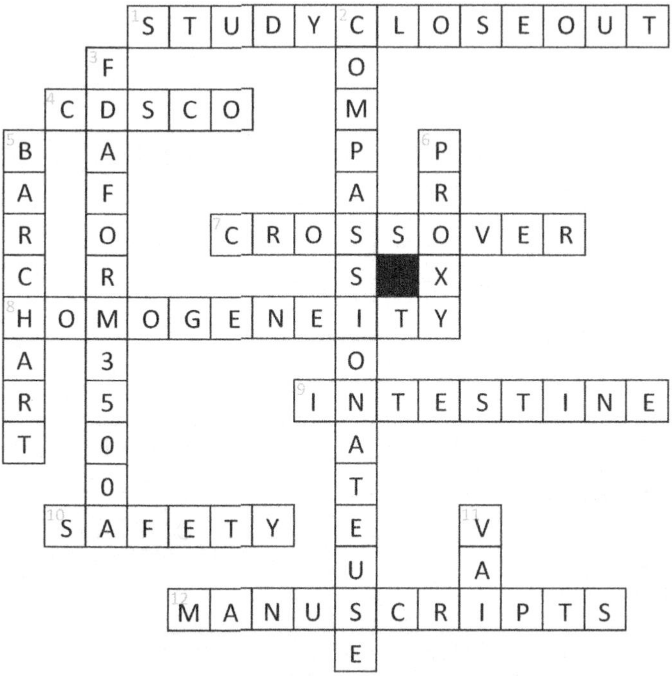

Across

1. STUDY CLOSEOUT
4. CDSCO
7. CROSS OVER
8. HOMOGENEITY
9. INTESTINE
10. SAFETY
12. MANUSCRIPTS

Down

2. COMPASSIONATE USE
3. FDA FORM 3500A
5. BAR CHART
6. PROXY
11. VAI

CDSCO: Central Drug Standard Control Organization; **VAI**: Voluntary Action Indicated

Crossword # 19

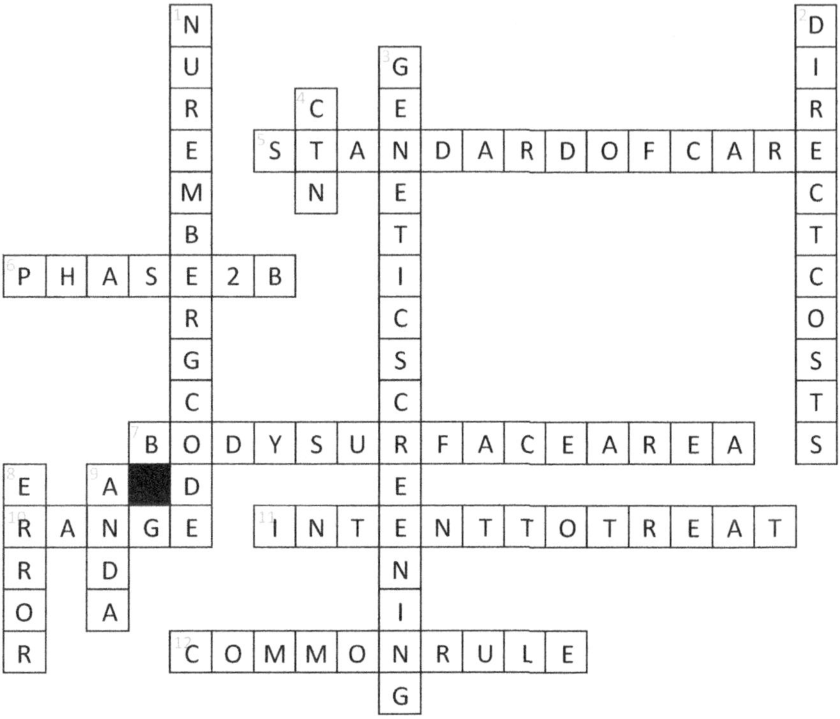

Across

5. STANDARD OF CARE
6. PHASE 2B
7. BODY SURFACE AREA
10. RANGE
11. INTENT TO TREAT
12. COMMON RULE

Down

1. NUREMBERG CODE
2. DIRECT COSTS
3. GENETIC SCREENING
4. CTN
8. ERROR
9. ANDA

CTN: Clinical Trial Notification; **ANDA**: Abbreviated New Drug Application

Crossword # 20

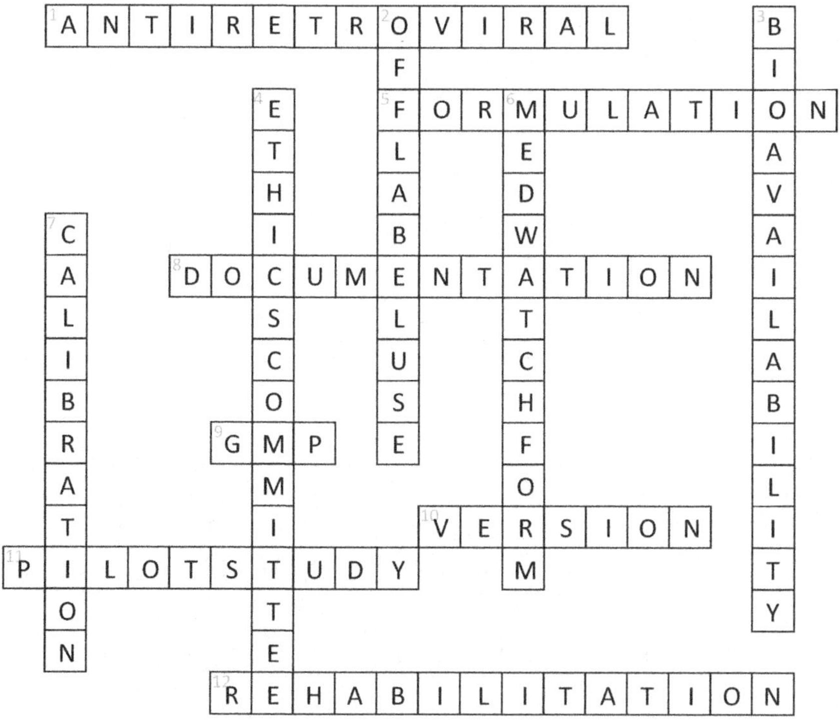

Across

1. ANTIRETROVIRAL
5. FORMULATION
8. DOCUMENTATION
9. GMP
10. VERSION
11. PILOT STUDY
12. REHABILITATION

Down

2. OFF LABEL USE
3. BIOAVAILABILITY
4. ETHICS COMMITTEE
6. MEDWATCH FORM
7. CALIBRATION

GMP: Good Manufacturing Practice

Crossword # 21

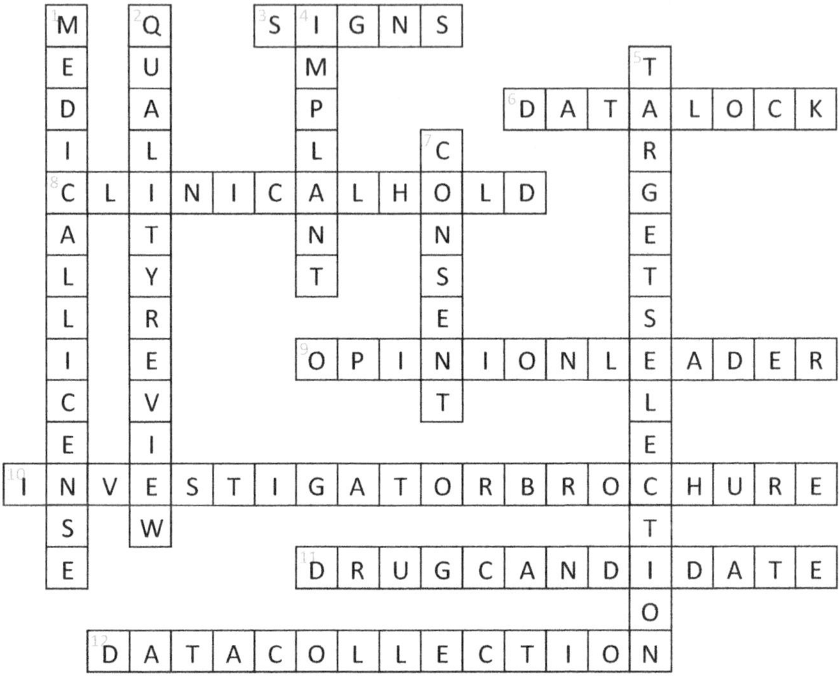

Across

3. SIGNS
6. DATA LOCK
8. CLINICAL HOLD
9. OPINION LEADER
10. INVESTIGATOR BROCHURE
11. DRUG CANDIDATE
12. DATA COLLECTION

Down

1. MEDICAL LICENSE
2. QUALITY REVIEW
4. IMPLANT
5. TARGET SELECTION
7. CONSENT

Crossword # 22

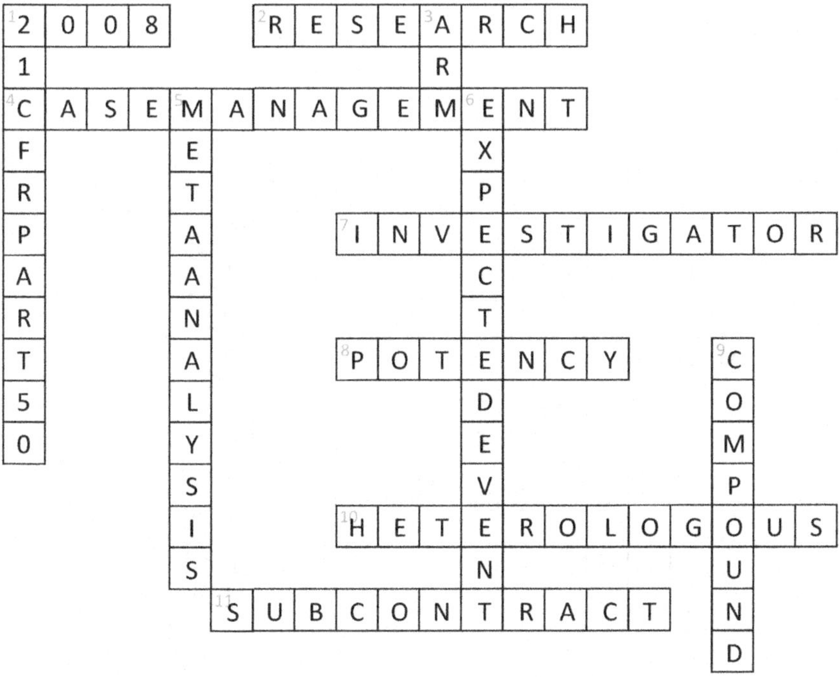

Across

1. 2008
2. RESEARCH
4. CASE MANAGEMENT
7. INVESTIGATOR
8. POTENCY
10. HETEROLOGOUS
11. SUBCONTRACT

Down

1. 21 CFR PART 50
3. ARM
5. META ANALYSIS
6. EXPECTED EVENT
9. COMPOUND

Crossword # 23

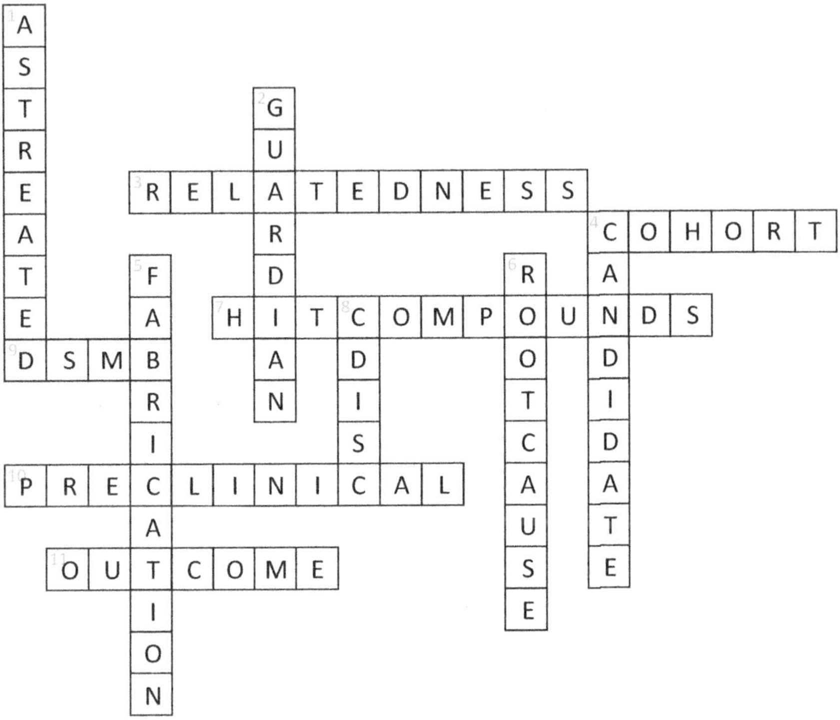

Across	**Down**
3. RELATEDNESS	1. AS TREATED
4. COHORT	2. GUARDIAN
7. HIT COMPOUNDS	4. CANDIDATE
9. DSMB	5. FABRICATION
10. PRE CLINICAL	6. ROOT CAUSE
11. OUTCOME	8. CDISC

DSMB: Data Safety Monitoring Board; **CDISC**: Clinical Data Interchange Standards Consortium

Crossword # 24

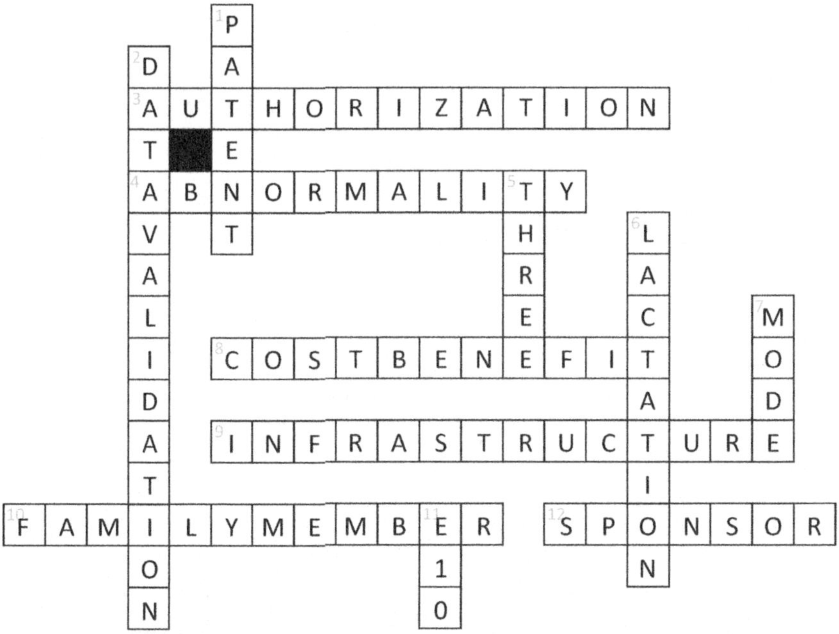

Across

3. AUTHORIZATION
4. ABNORMALITY
8. COST BENEFIT
9. INFRASTRUCTURE
10. FAMILY MEMBER
12. SPONSOR

Down

1. PATENT
2. DATA VALIDATION
5. THREE
6. LACTATION
7. MODE
11. E10

Crossword # 25

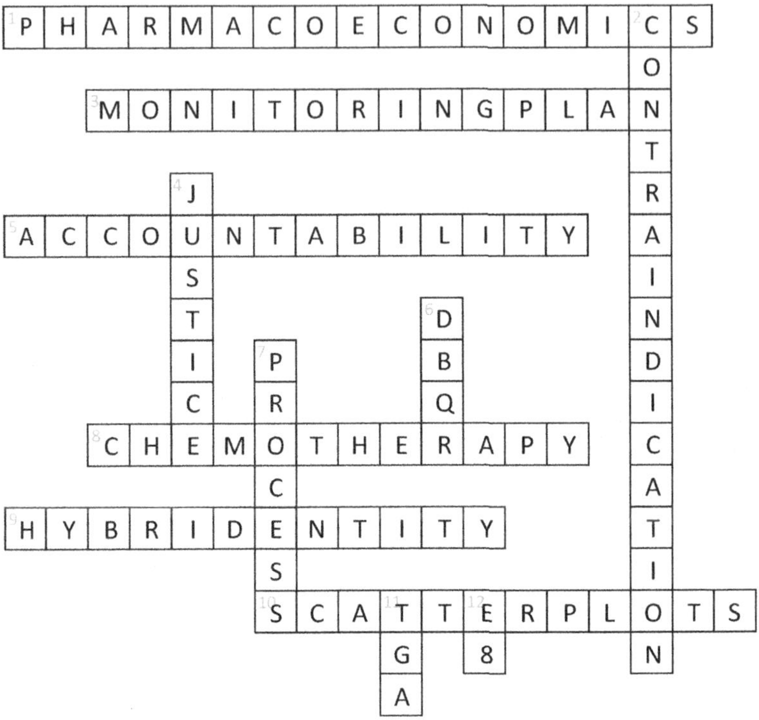

Across

1. PHARMACOECONOMICS
3. MONITORING PLAN
5. ACCOUNTABILITY
8. CHEMOTHERAPY
9. HYBRIDENTITY
10. SCATTER PLOTS

Down

2. CONTRAINDICATION
4. JUSTICE
6. DBQR
7. PROCESS
11. TGA
12. E8

DBQR: Database Quality Review; **TGA**: Therapeutics Goods Administration

Crossword # 26

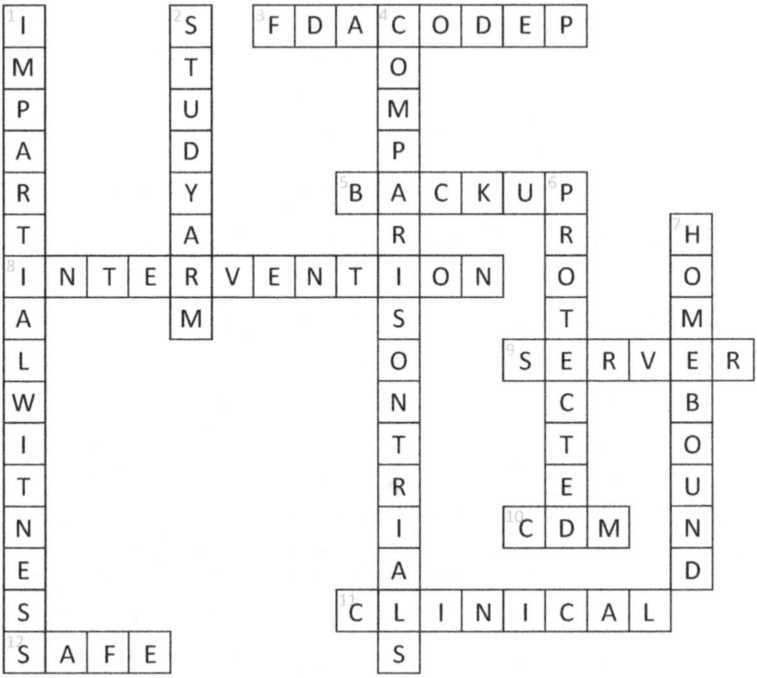

Across

3. FDA CODE P
5. BACK UP
8. INTERVENTION
9. SERVER
10. CDM
11. CLINICAL
12. SAFE

Down

1. IMPARTIAL WITNESS
2. STUDY ARM
4. COMPARISON TRIALS
6. PROTECTED
7. HOME BOUND

CDM: Clinical Data Manager

Crossword # 27

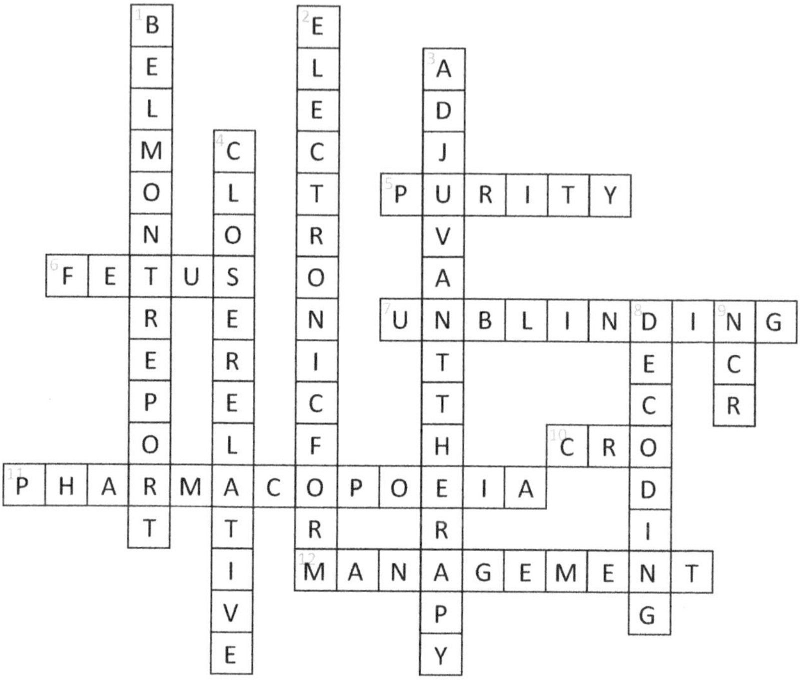

Across

5. PURITY
6. FETUS
7. UNBLINDING
10. CRO
11. PHARMACOPOEIA
12. MANAGEMENT

Down

1. BELMONT REPORT
2. ELECTRONIC FORM
3. ADJUVANT THERAPY
4. CLOSE RELATIVE
8. DECODING
9. NCR

CRO: Contract Research Organization; **NCR**: No Carbon Required

Crossword # 28

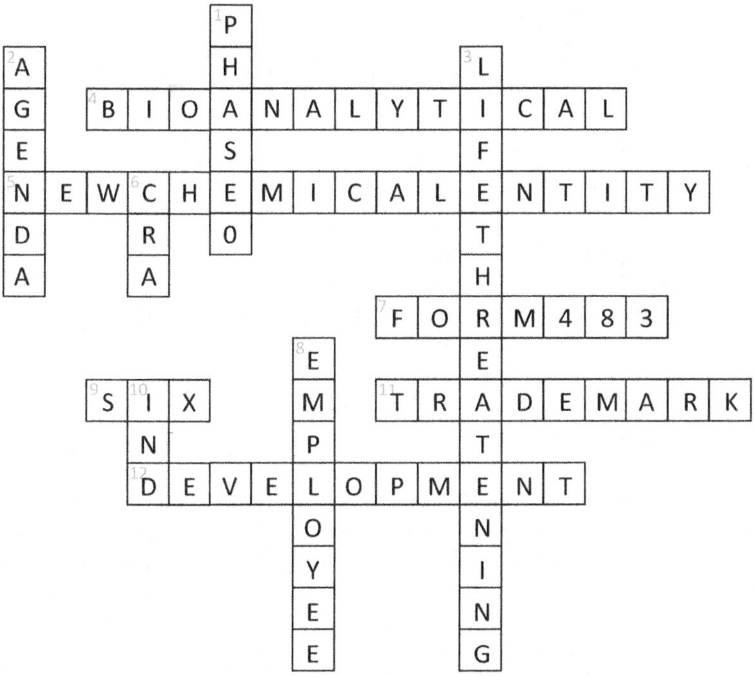

Across

4. BIO ANALYTICAL
5. NEW CHEMICAL ENTITY
7. FORM 483
9. SIX
11. TRADE MARK
12. DEVELOPMENT

Down

1. PHASE 0
2. AGENDA
3. LIFE THREATENING
6. CRA
8. EMPLOYEE
10. IND

CRA: Clinical Research Associate; **IND**: Investigational New Drug

Crossword # 29

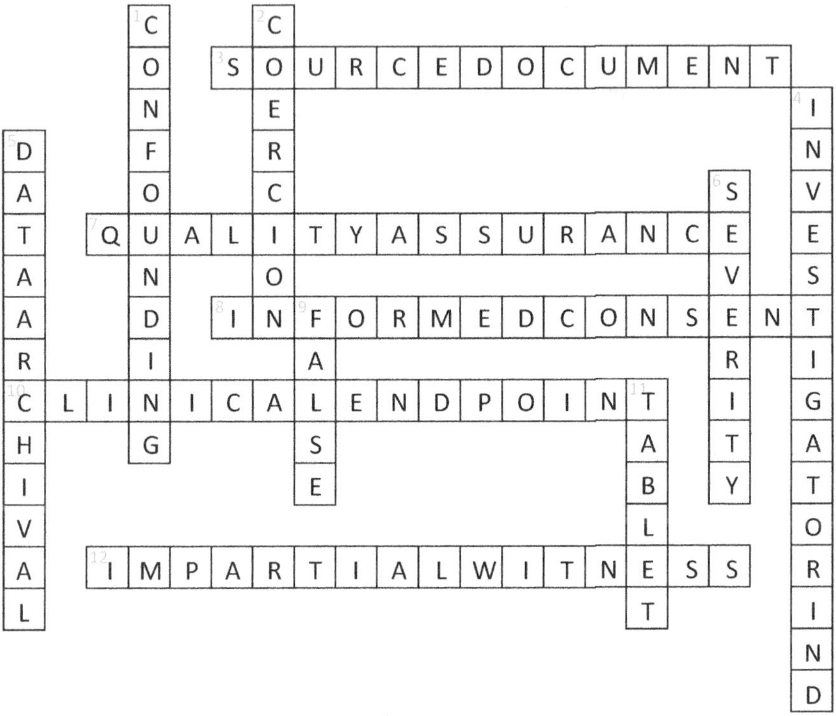

Across

3. SOURCE DOCUMENT
7. QUALITY ASSURANCE
8. INFORMED CONSENT
10. CLINICAL ENDPOINT
12. IMPARTIAL WITNESS

Down

1. CONFOUNDING
2. COERCION
4. INVESTIGATOR IND
5. DATA ARCHIVAL
6. SEVERITY
9. FALSE
11. TABLET

Crossword # 30

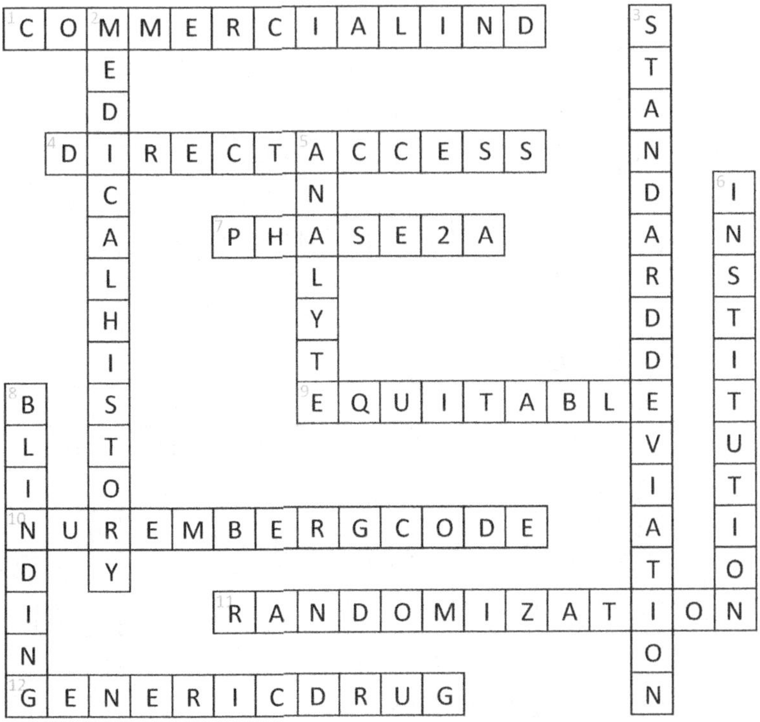

Across

1. COMMERCIAL IND
4. DIRECT ACCESS
7. PHASE 2A
9. EQUITABLE
10. NUREMBERG CODE
11. RANDOMIZATION
12. GENERIC DRUG

Down

2. MEDICAL HISTORY
3. STANDARD DEVIATION
5. ANALYTE
6. INSTITUTION
8. BLINDING

Crossword # 31

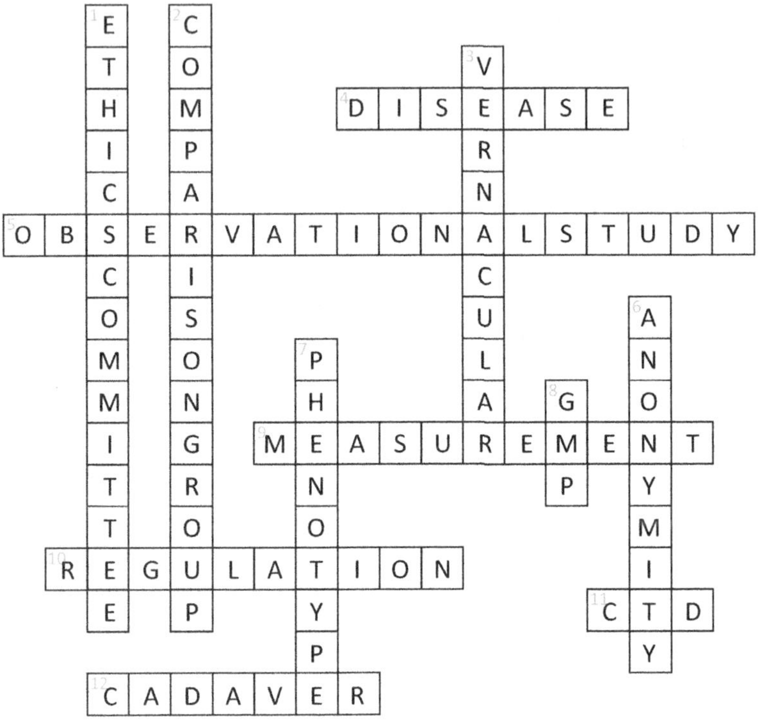

Across

4. DISEASE
5. OBSERVATIONAL STUDY
9. MEASUREMENT
10. REGULATION
11. CTD
12. CADAVER

Down

1. ETHICS COMMITTEE
2. COMPARISON GROUP
3. VERNACULAR
6. ANONYMITY
7. PHENOTYPE
8. GMP

CTD: Common Technical Document; **GMP**: Good Manufacturing Practice

Crossword # 32

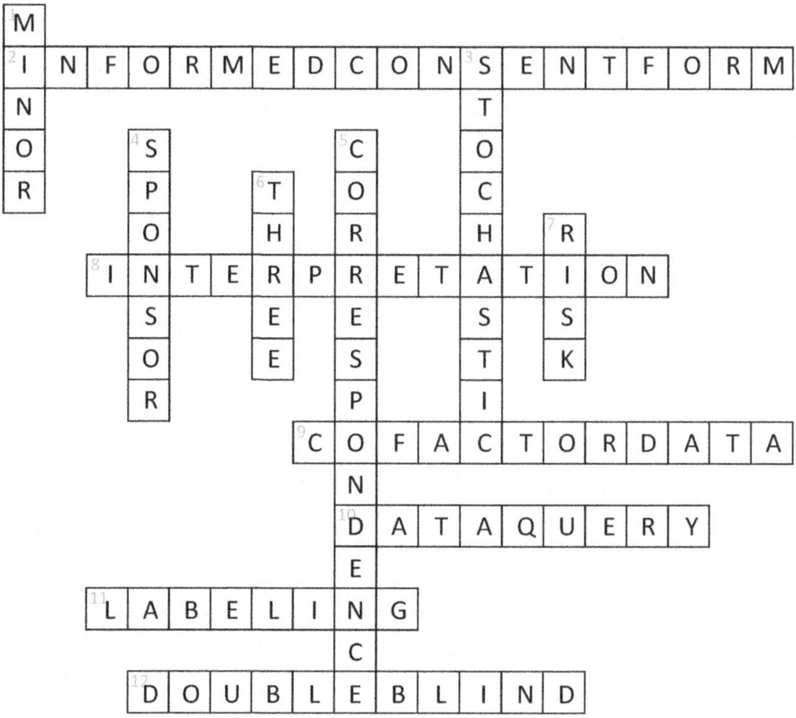

Across		**Down**	
2.	INFORMED CONSENT FORM	1.	MINOR
8.	INTERPRETATION	3.	STOCHASTIC
9.	COFACTOR DATA	4.	SPONSOR
10.	DATA QUERY	5.	CORRESPONDENCE
11.	LABELING	6.	THREE
12.	DOUBLE BLIND	7.	RISK

Crossword # 33

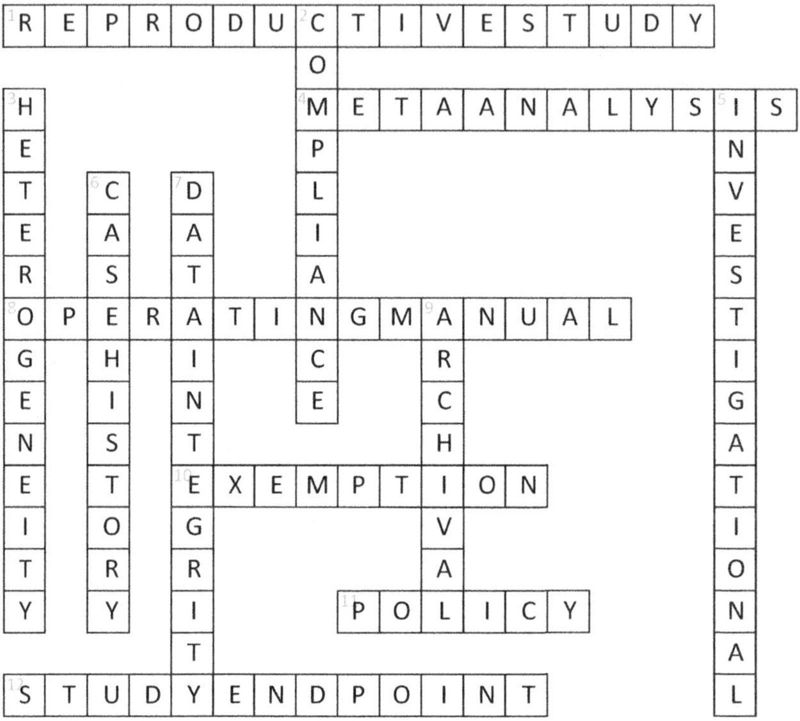

Across

1. REPRODUCTIVE STUDY
4. META ANALYSIS
8. OPERATING MANUAL
10. EXEMPTION
11. POLICY
12. STUDY ENDPOINT

Down

2. COMPLIANCE
3. HETEROGENEITY
5. INVESTIGATIONAL
6. CASE HISTORY
7. DATA INTEGRITY
9. ARCHIVAL

Crossword # 34

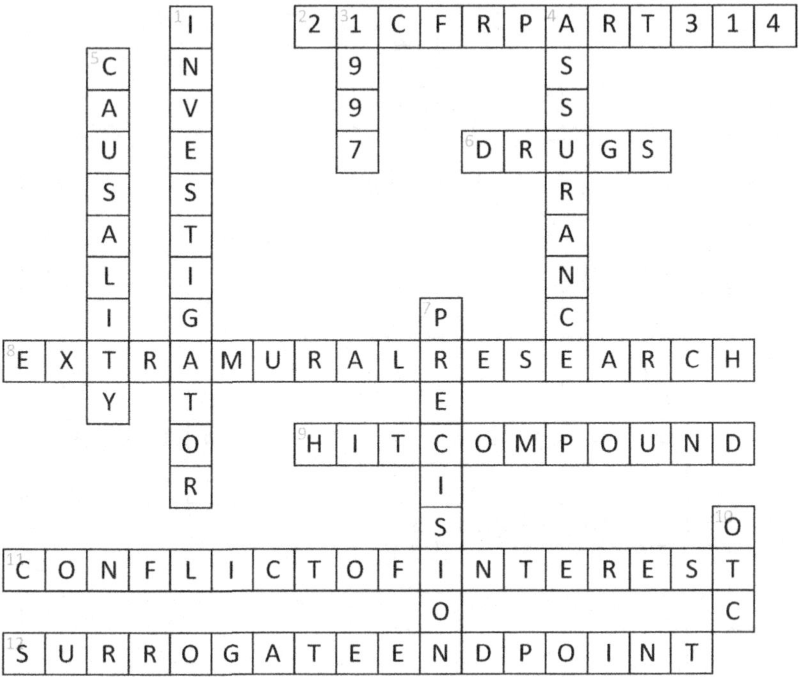

Across

2. 21 CFR PART 314
6. DRUGS
8. EXTRAMURAL RESEARCH
9. HIT COMPOUND
11. CONFLICT OF INTEREST
12. SURROGATE ENDPOINT

Down

1. INVESTIGATOR
3. 1997
4. ASSURANCE
5. CAUSALITY
7. PRECISION
10. OTC

OTC: Over The Counter

Crossword # 35

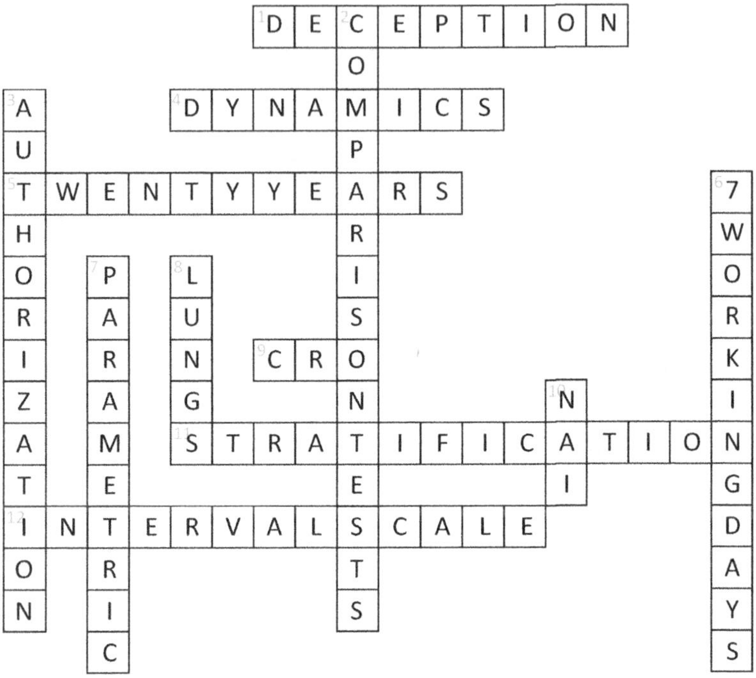

Across

1. DECEPTION
4. DYNAMICS
5. TWENTY YEARS
9. CRO
11. STRATIFICATION
12. INTERVAL SCALE

Down

2. COMPARISON TESTS
3. AUTHORIZATION
6. 7 WORKING DAYS
7. PARAMETRIC
8. LUNGS
10. NAI

CRO: Contract Research Organization; **NAI**: No Action Indicated

Crossword # 36

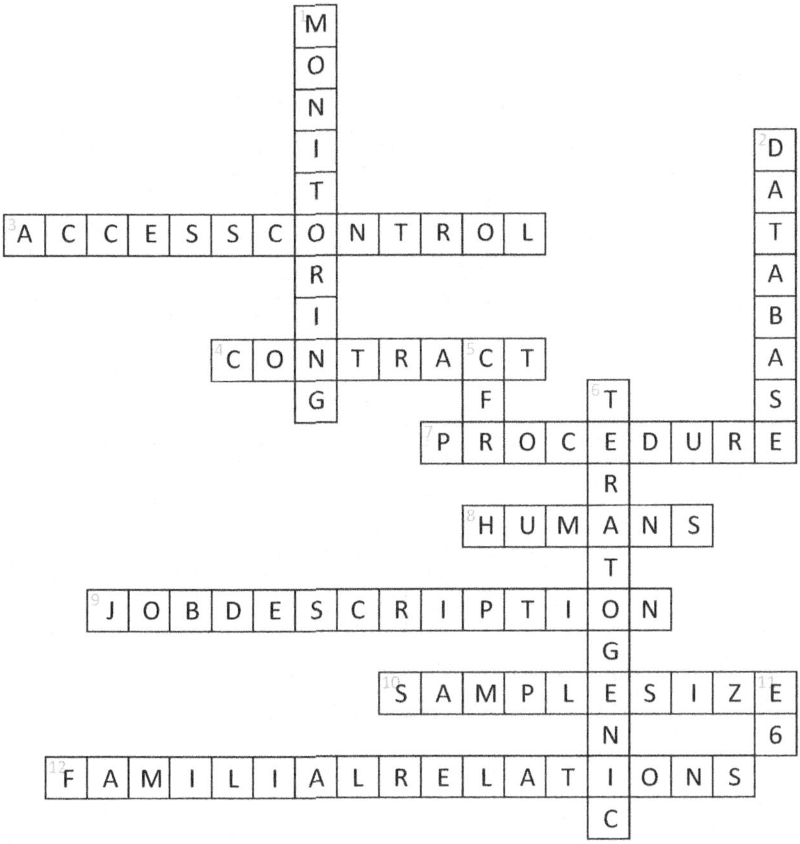

Across

3. ACCESS CONTROL
4. CONTRACT
7. PROCEDURE
8. HUMANS
9. JOB DESCRIPTION
10. SAMPLE SIZE
12. FAMILIAL RELATIONS

Down

1. MONITORING
2. DATABASE
5. CFR
6. TERATOGENIC
11. E6

Crossword # 37

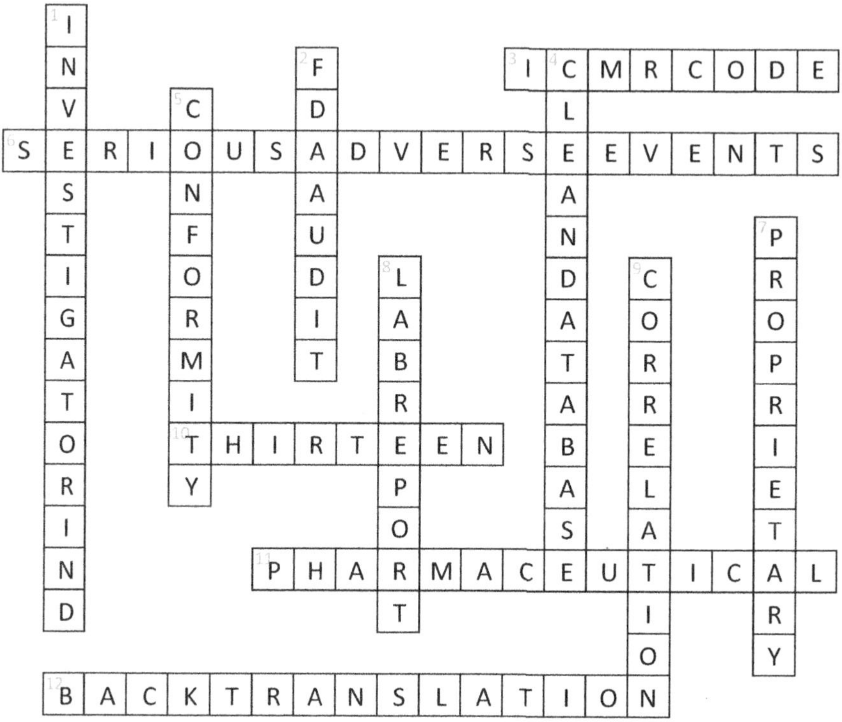

Across

3. ICMR CODE
6. SERIOUS ADVERSE EVENTS
10. THIRTEEN
11. PHARMACEUTICAL
12. BACK TRANSLATION

Down

1. INVESTIGATOR IND
2. FDA AUDIT
4. CLEAN DATABASE
5. CONFORMITY
7. PROPRIETARY
8. LAB REPORT
9. CORRELATION

Crossword # 38

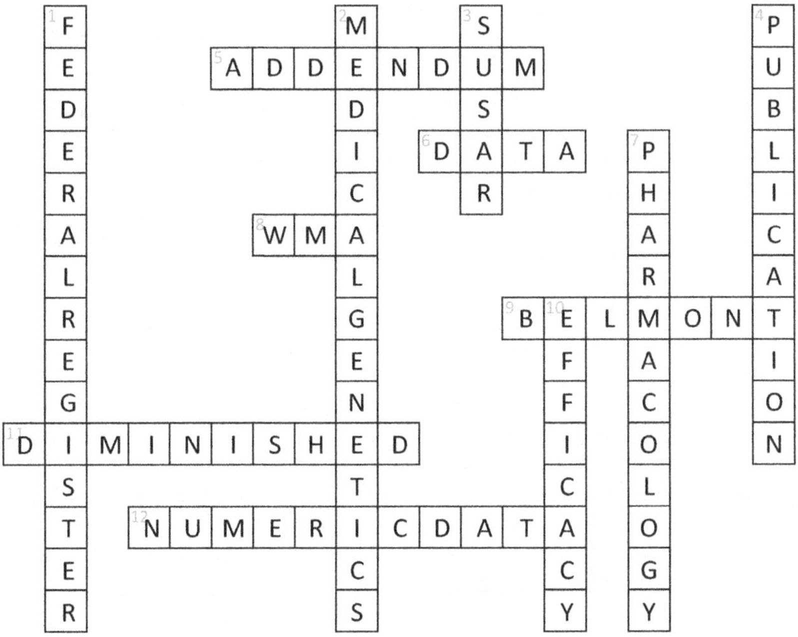

Across

5. ADDENDUM
6. DATA
8. WMA
9. BELMONT
11. DIMINISHED
12. NUMERIC DATA

Down

1. FEDERAL REGISTER
2. MEDICAL GENETICS
3. SUSAR
4. PUBLICATION
7. PHARMACOLOGY
10. EFFICACY

WMA: World Medical Association; **SUSAR**: Suspected Unexpected Serious Adverse Reaction

Crossword # 39

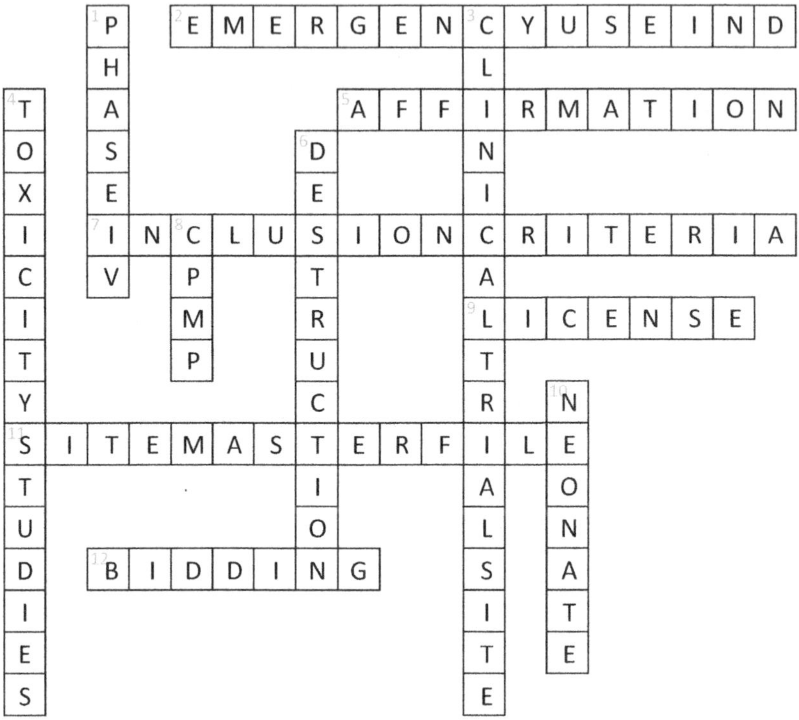

Across		**Down**	
2.	EMERGENCY USE IND	1.	PHASE IV
5.	AFFIRMATION	3.	CLINICAL TRIAL SITE
7.	INCLUSION CRITERIA	4.	TOXICITY STUDIES
9.	LICENSE	6.	DESTRUCTION
11.	SITE MASTER FILE	8.	CPMP
12.	BIDDING	10.	NEONATE

CPMP: Committee for Proprietary Medicinal Products

Crossword # 40

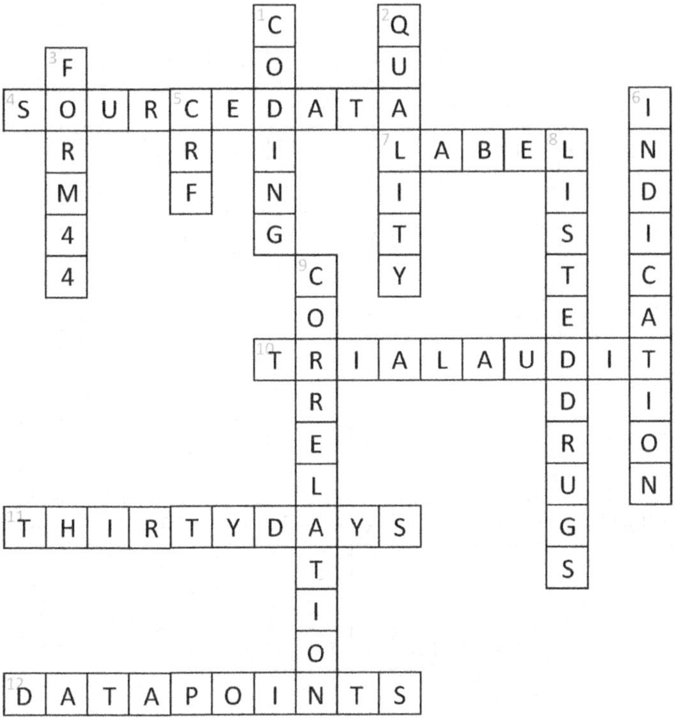

Across

4. SOURCE DATA
7. LABEL
10. TRIAL AUDIT
11. THIRTY DAYS
12. DATA POINTS

Down

1. CODING
2. QUALITY
3. FORM 44
5. CRF
6. INDICATION
8. LISTED DRUGS
9. CORRELATION

CRF: Case Report Form

Crossword # 41

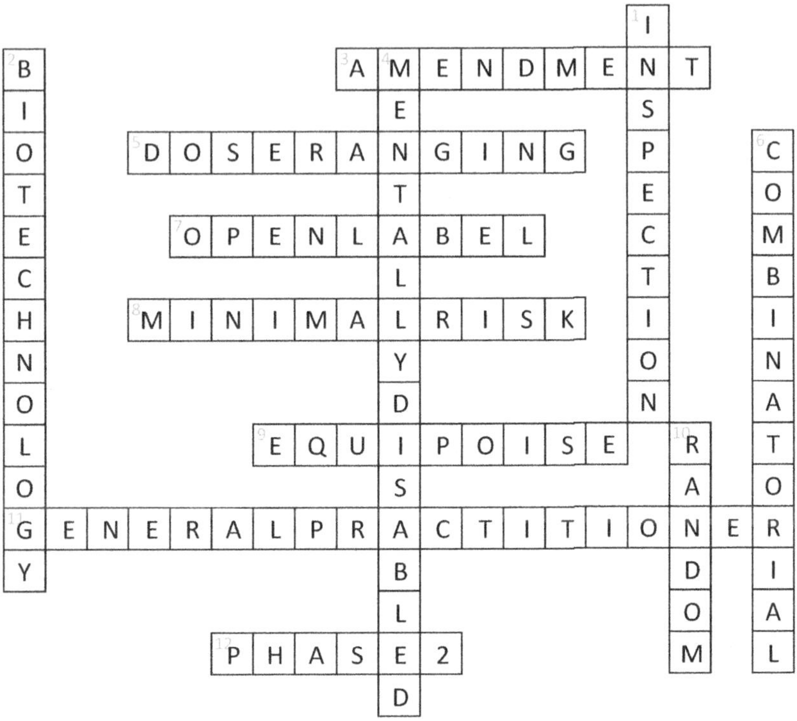

Across

3. AMENDMENT
5. DOSE RANGING
7. OPEN LABEL
8. MINIMAL RISK
9. EQUIPOISE
11. GENERAL PRACTITIONER
12. PHASE 2

Down

1. INSPECTION
2. BIOTECHNOLOGY
4. MENTALLY DISABLED
6. COMBINATORIAL
10. RANDOM

Crossword # 42

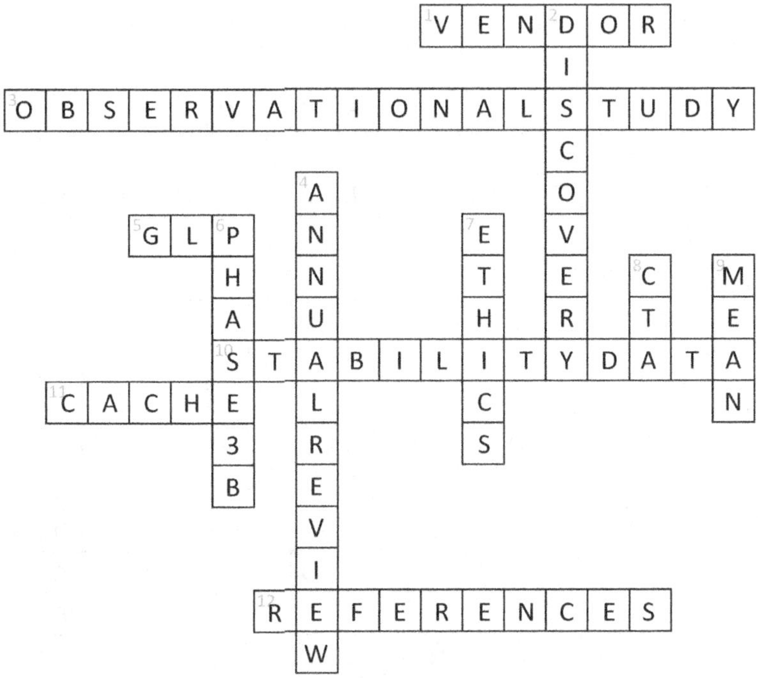

Across

1. VENDOR
3. OBSERVATIONAL STUDY
5. GLP
10. STABILITY DATA
11. CACHE
12. REFERENCES

Down

2. DISCOVERY
4. ANNUAL REVIEW
6. PHASE 3B
7. ETHICS
8. CTA
9. MEAN

GLP: Good Laboratory Practice; **CTA**: Clinical Trial Agreement

Crossword # 43

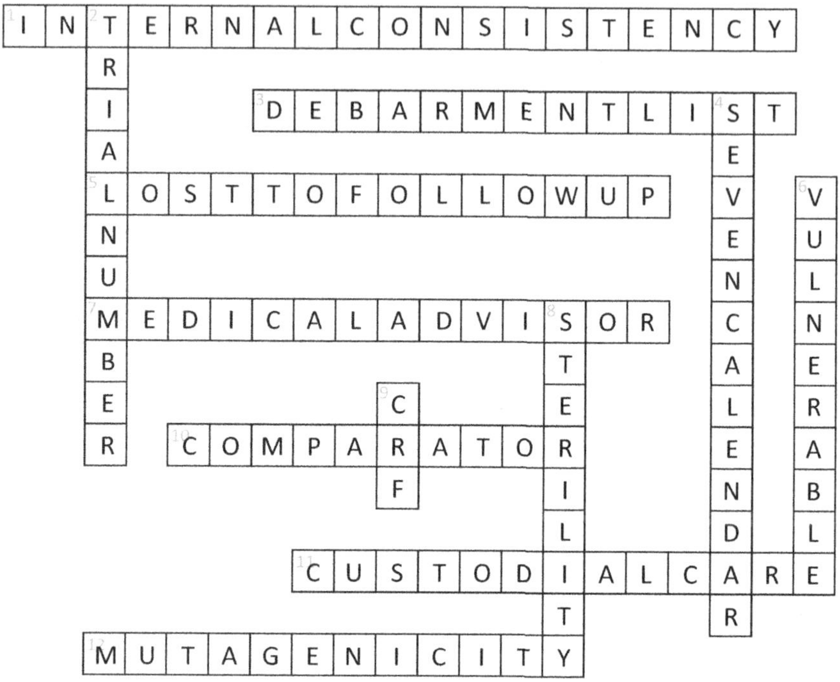

Across

1. INTERNAL CONSISTENCY
3. DEBARMENT LIST
5. LOST TO FOLLOW UP
7. MEDICAL ADVISOR
10. COMPARATOR
11. CUSTODIAL CARE
12. MUTAGENICITY

Down

2. TRIAL NUMBER
4. SEVEN CALENDAR
6. VULNERABLE
8. STERILITY
9. CRF

CRF: Case Report Form

Crossword # 44

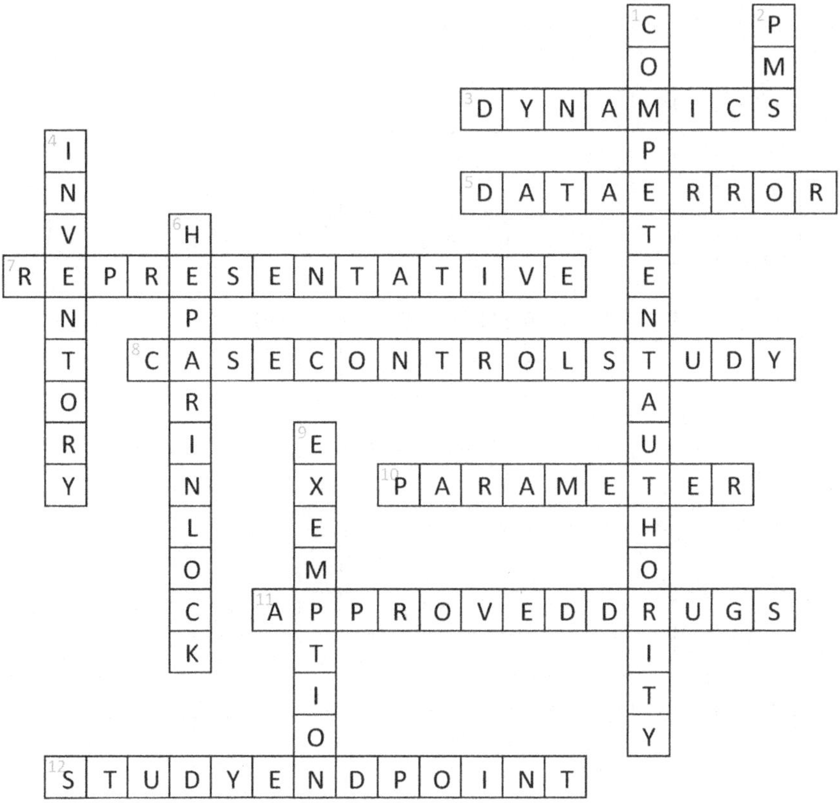

Across

3. DYNAMICS
5. DATA ERROR
7. REPRESENTATIVE
8. CASE CONTROL STUDY
10. PARAMETER
11. APPROVED DRUGS
12. STUDY ENDPOINT

Down

1. COMPETENT AUTHORITY
2. PMS
4. INVENTORY
6. HEPARIN LOCK
9. EXEMPTION

PMS: Post Marketing Surveillance

Crossword # 45

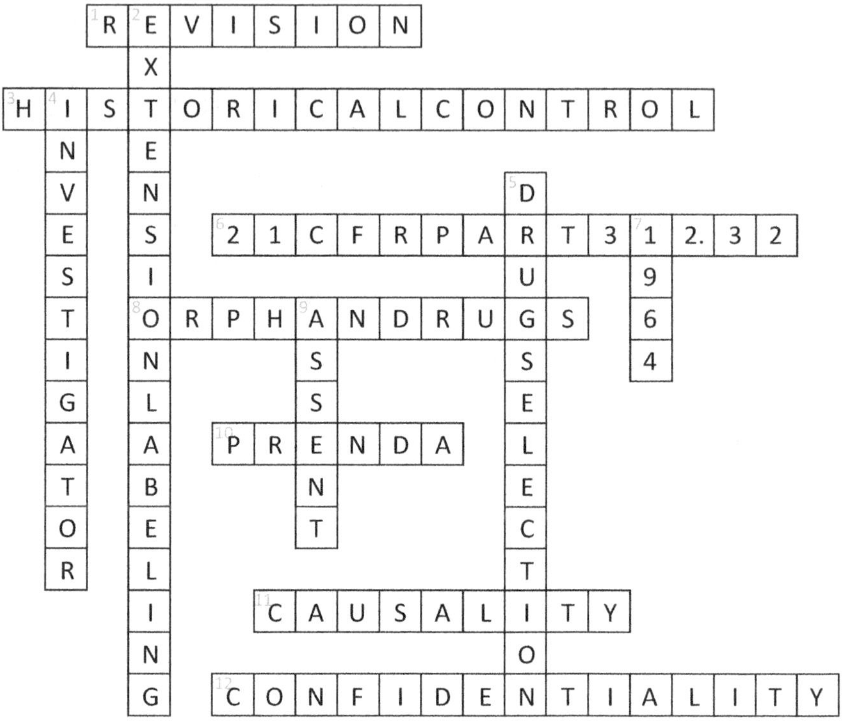

Across

1. REVISION
3. HISTORICAL CONTROL
6. 21 CFR PART 312.32
8. ORPHAN DRUGS
10. PRE NDA
11. CAUSALITY
12. CONFIDENTIALITY

Down

2. EXTENSION LABELING
4. INVESTIGATOR
5. DRUG SELECTION
7. 1964
9. ASSENT

NDA: New Drug Application

Crossword # 46

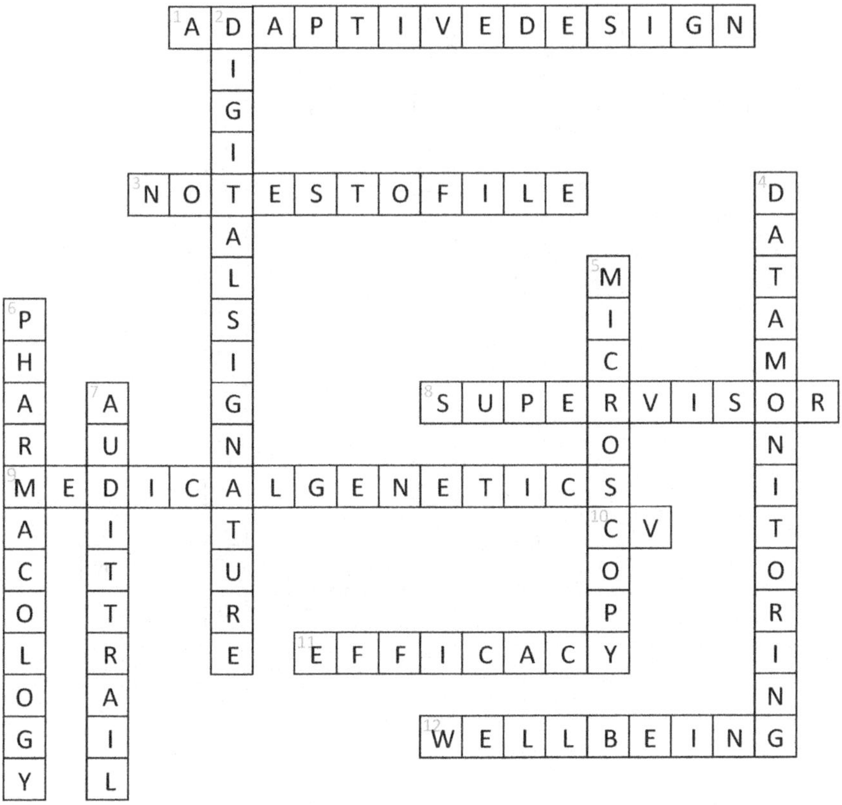

Across

1. ADAPTIVE DESIGN
3. NOTES TO FILE
8. SUPERVISOR
9. MEDICAL GENETICS
10. CV
11. EFFICACY
12. WELL BEING

Down

2. DIGITAL SIGNATURE
4. DATA MONITORING
5. MICROSCOPY
6. PHARMACOLOGY
7. AUDIT TRAIL

CV: Curriculum Vitae

Crossword # 47

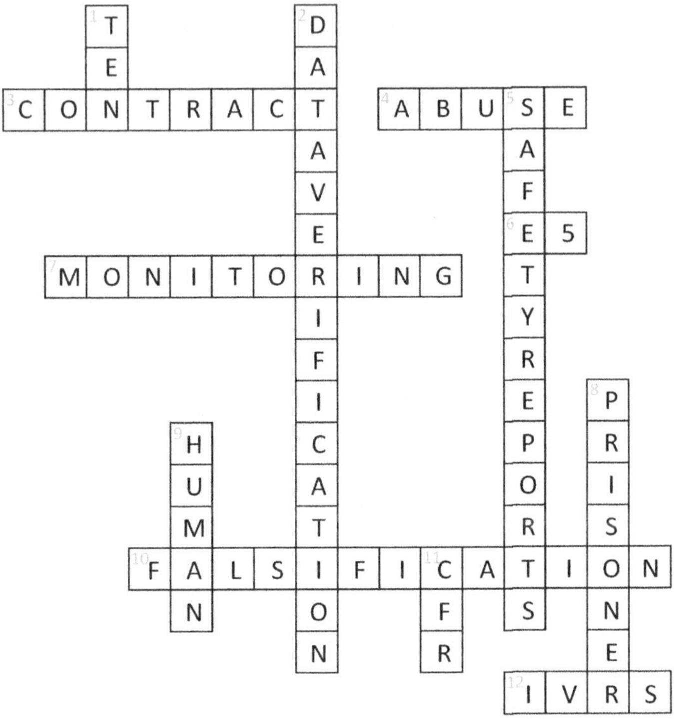

Across

3. CONTRACT
4. ABUSE
6. E5
7. MONITORING
10. FALSIFICATION
12. IVRS

Down

1. TEN
2. DATA VERIFICATION
5. SAFETY REPORTS
8. PRISONER
9. HUMAN
11. CFR

IVRS: Interactive Voice Response System; **CFR**: Code of Federal Regulations

Crossword # 48

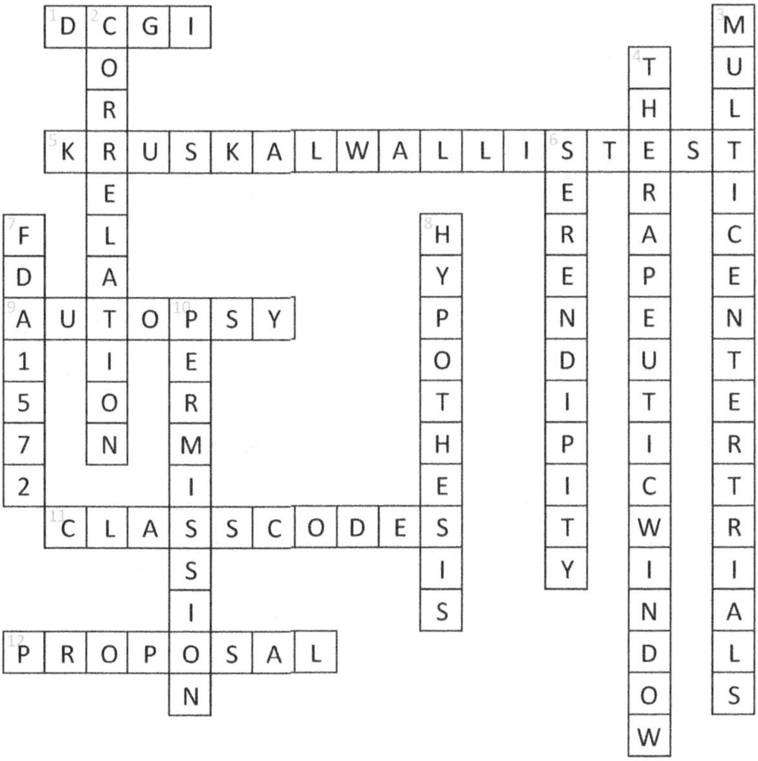

Across

1. DCGI
5. KRUSKAL WALLIS TEST
9. AUTOPSY
11. CLASS CODES
12. PROPOSAL

Down

2. CORRELATION
3. MULTICENTER TRIALS
4. THERAPEUTIC WINDOW
6. SERENDIPITY
7. FDA 1572
8. HYPOTHESIS
10. PERMISSION

DCGI: Drug Controller General of India

Crossword # 49

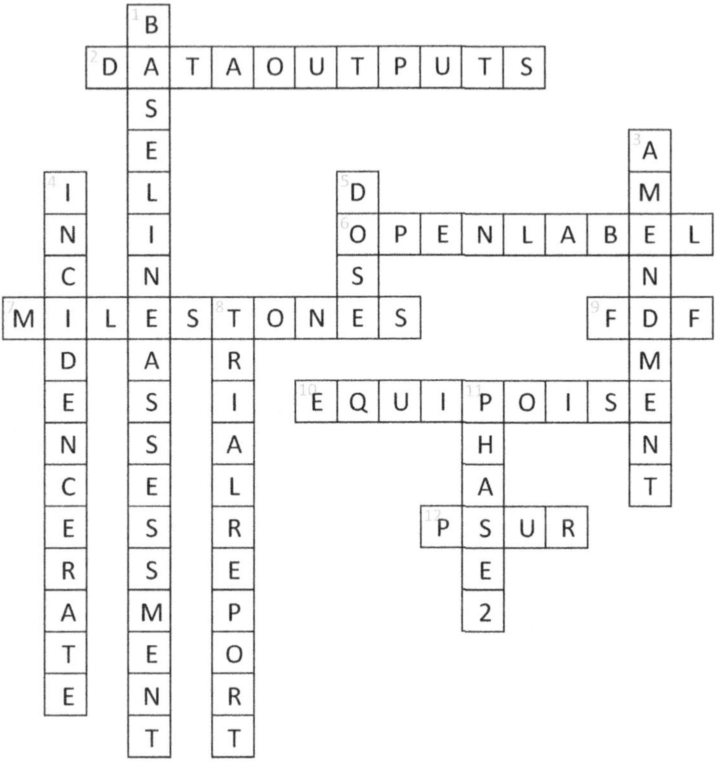

Across

2. DATA OUTPUTS
6. OPEN LABEL
7. MILESTONES
9. FDF
10. EQUIPOISE
12. PSUR

Down

1. BASELINE ASSESSMENT
3. AMENDMENT
4. INCIDENCE RATE
5. DOSE
8. TRIAL REPORT
11. PHASE 2

FDF: Financial Disclosure Form; **PSUR**: Periodic Safety Update Report

Crossword # 50

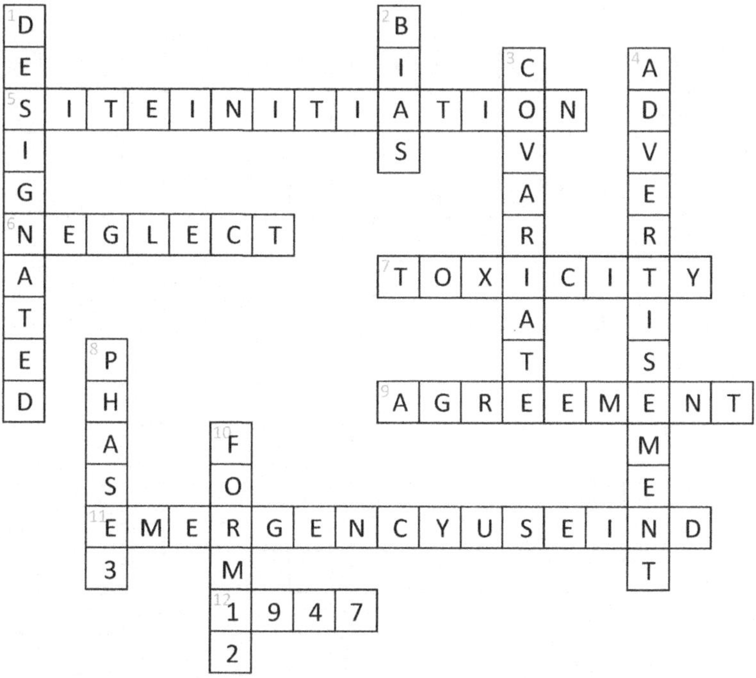

Across

5. SITE INITIATION
6. NEGLECT
7. TOXICITY
9. AGREEMENT
11. EMERGENCY USE IND
12. 1947

Down

1. DESIGNATED
2. BIAS
3. COVARIATE
4. ADVERTISEMENT
8. PHASE 3
10. FORM 12

Crossword # 51

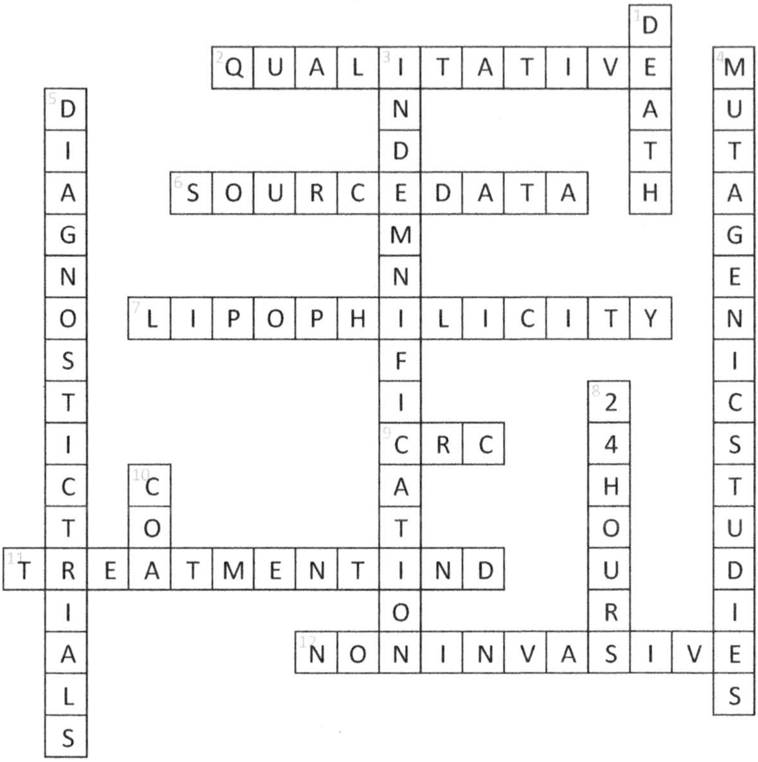

Across

2. QUALITATIVE
6. SOURCE DATA
7. LIPOPHILICITY
9. CRC
11. TREATMENT IND
12. NON INVASIVE

Down

1. DEATH
3. INDEMNIFICATION
4. MUTAGENIC STUDIES
5. DIAGNOSTIC TRIALS
8. 24 HOURS
10. COA

CRC: Clinical Research Coordinator

Crossword # 52

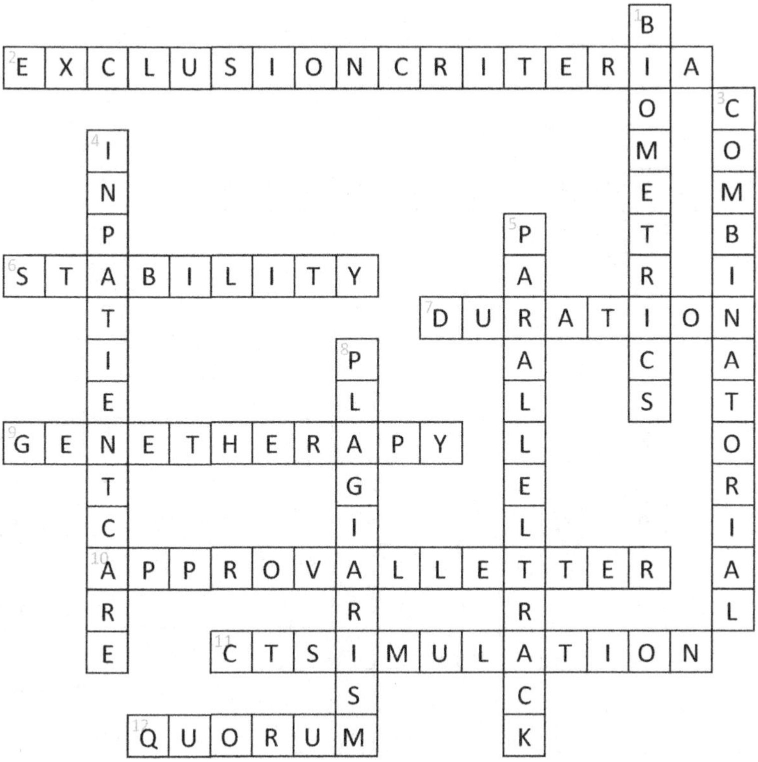

Across

2. EXCLUSION CRITERIA
6. STABILITY
7. DURATION
9. GENE THERAPY
10. APPROVAL LETTER
11. CT SIMULATION
12. QUORUM

Down

1. BIOMETRICS
3. COMBINATORIAL
4. INPATIENT CARE
5. PARALLEL TRACK
8. PLAGIARISM

Crossword # 53

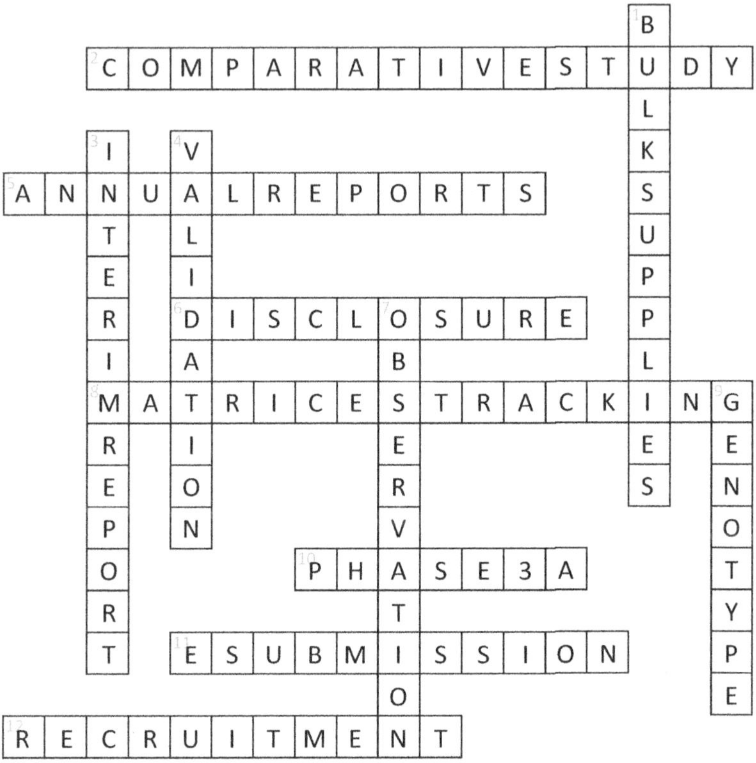

Across

2. COMPARATIVE STUDY
5. ANNUAL REPORTS
6. DISCLOSURE
8. MATRICES TRACKING
10. PHASE 3A
11. e SUBMISSION
12. RECRUITMENT

Down

1. BULK SUPPLIES
3. INTERIM REPORT
4. VALIDATION
7. OBSERVATION
9. GENOTYPE

Crossword # 54

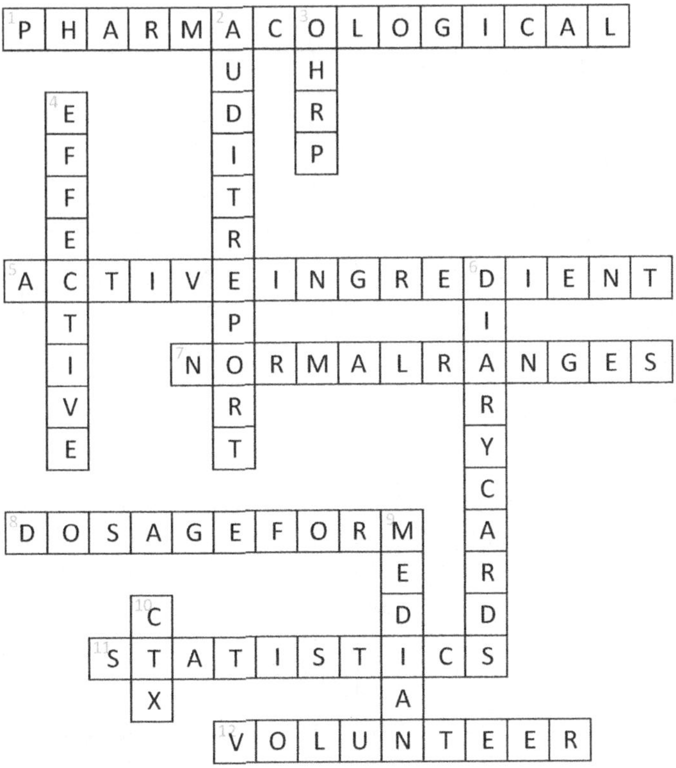

Across

1. PHARMACOLOGICAL
5. ACTIVE INGREDIENT
7. NORMAL RANGES
8. DOSAGE FORM
11. STATISTICS
12. VOLUNTEER

Down

2. AUDIT REPORT
3. OHRP
4. EFFECTIVE
6. DIARY CARDS
9. MEDIAN
10. CTX

OHRP: Office for Human Research Protection

Crossword # 55

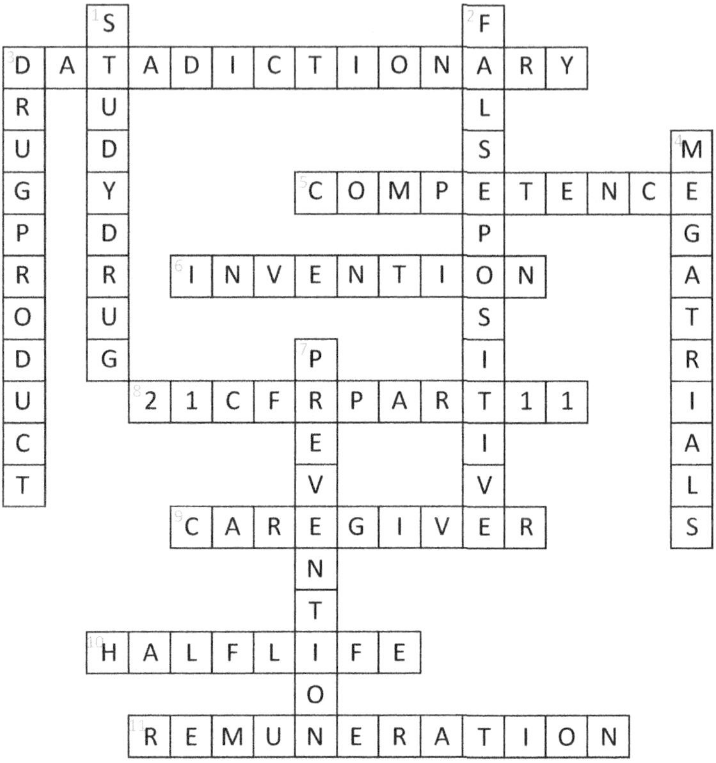

Across

3. DATA DICTIONARY
5. COMPETENCE
6. INVENTION
8. 21 CFR PART 11
9. CAREGIVER
10. HALF LIFE
11. REMUNERATION

Down

1. STUDY DRUG
2. FALSE POSITIVE
3. DRUG PRODUCT
4. MEGA TRIALS
7. PREVENTION

Crossword # 56

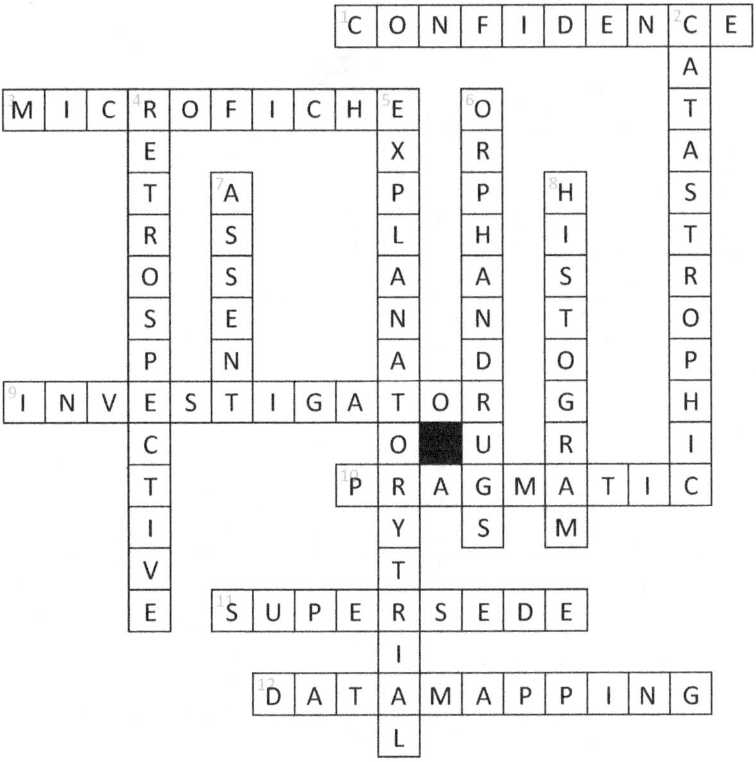

Across

1. CONFIDENCE
3. MICROFICHE
9. INVESTIGATOR
10. PRAGMATIC
11. SUPERSEDE
12. DATA MAPPING

Down

2. CATASTROPHIC
4. RETROSPECTIVE
5. EXPLANATORY TRIAL
6. ORPHAN DRUGS
7. ASSENT
8. HISTOGRAM

Crossword # 57

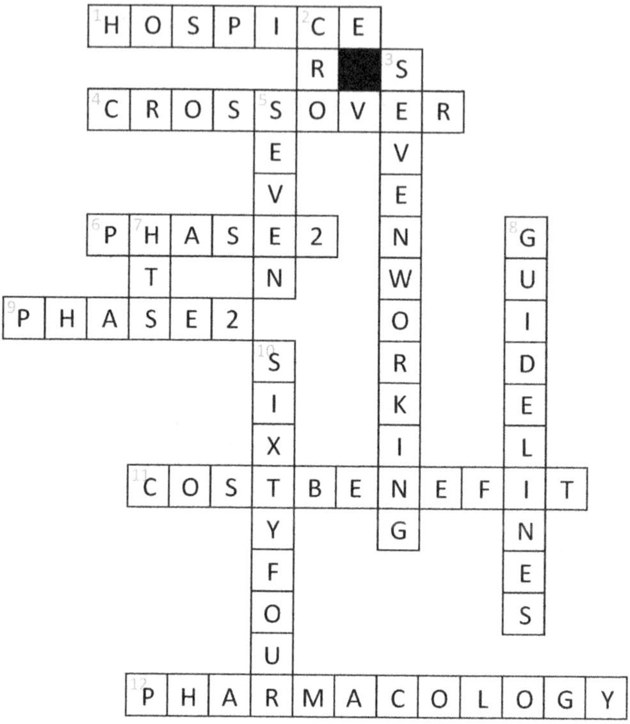

Across

1. HOSPICE
4. CROSSOVER
6. PHASE 2
9. PHASE 2
11. COST BENEFIT
12. PHARMACOLOGY

Down

2. CRO
3. SEVEN WORKING
5. SEVEN
7. HTS
8. GUIDELINES
10. SIXTY FOUR

CRO: Contract Research Organization; **HTS**: High Throughput Screening

Crossword # 58

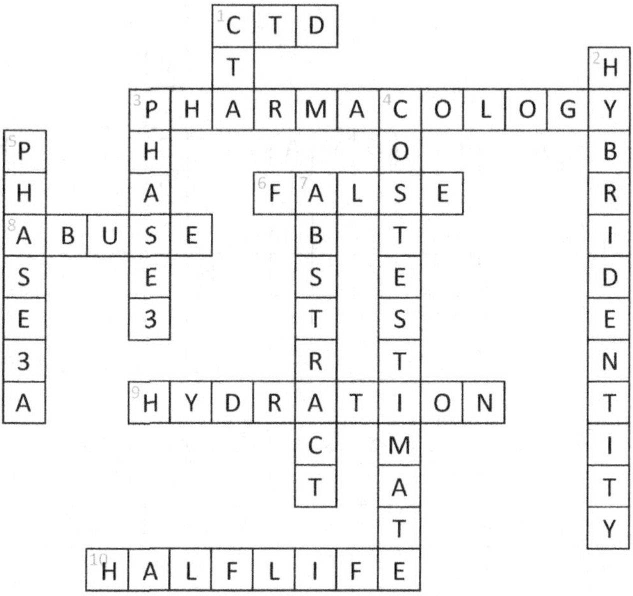

Across

1. CTD
3. PHARMACOLOGY
6. FALSE
8. ABUSE
9. HYDRATION
10. HALF LIFE

Down

1. CTA
2. HYBRID ENTITY
3. PHASE 3
4. COST ESTIMATE
5. PHASE 3A
7. ABSTRACT

CTD: Common Technical Document; **CTA**: Clinical Trial Agreement

Crossword # 59

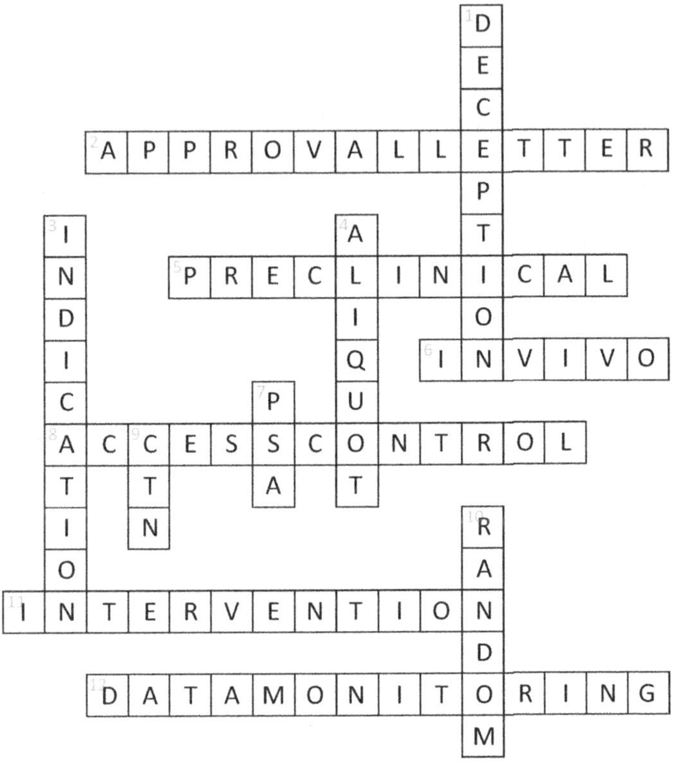

Across

2. APPROVAL LETTER
5. PRE CLINICAL
6. IN VIVO
8. ACCESS CONTROL
11. INTERVENTION
12. DATA MONITORING

Down

1. DECEPTION
3. INDICATION
4. ALIQUOT
7. PSA
9. CTN
10. RANDOM

PSA: Professional Services Agreement; **CTN**: Clinical Trial Notification

Crossword # 60

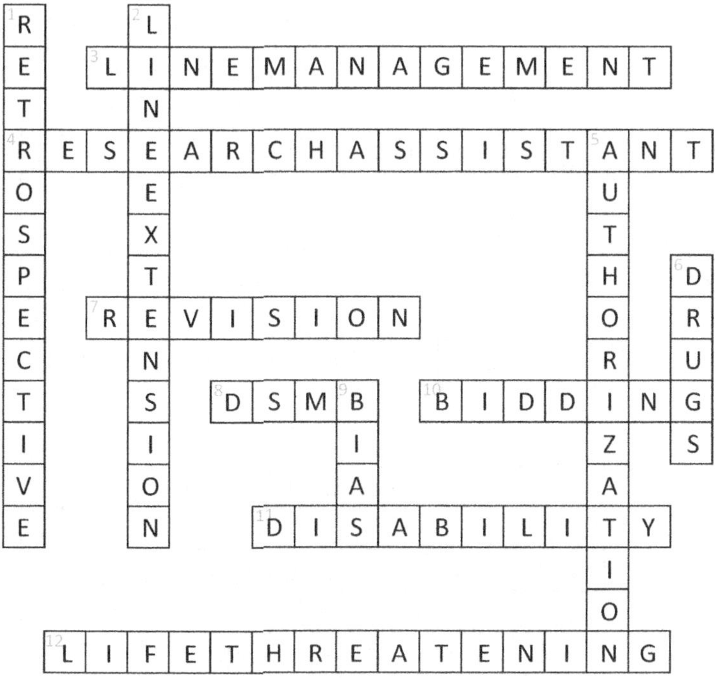

Across

3. LINE MANAGEMENT
4. RESEARCH ASSISTANT
7. REVISION
8. DSMB
10. BIDDING
11. DISABILITY
12. LIFE THREATENING

Down

1. RETROSPECTIVE
2. LINE EXTENSION
5. AUTHORIZATION
6. DRUGS
9. BIAS

DSMB: Data Safety Monitoring Board

Crossword # 61

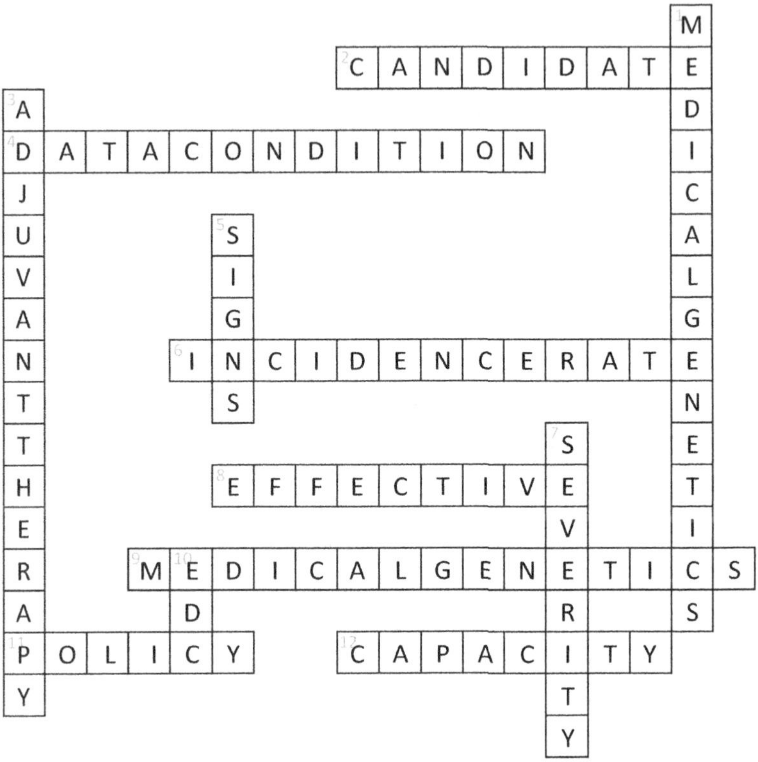

Across

2. CANDIDATE
4. DATA CONDITION
6. INCIDENCE RATE
8. EFFECTIVE
9. MEDICAL GENETICS
11. POLICY
12. CAPACITY

Down

1. MEDICAL GENETICS
3. ADJUVANT THERAPY
5. SIGNS
7. SEVERITY
10. EDC

EDC: Electronic Data Capture

Crossword # 62

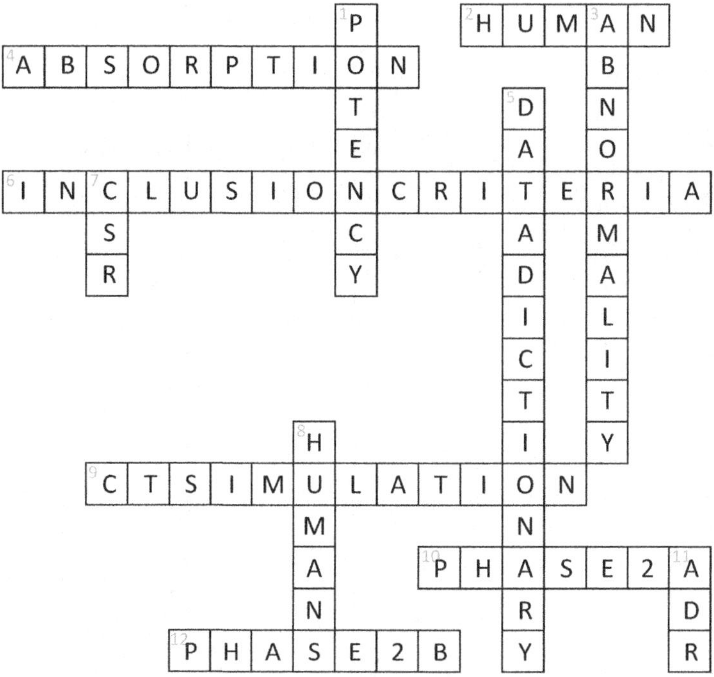

Across

2. HUMAN
4. ABSORPTION
6. INCLUSION CRITERIA
9. CT SIMULATION
10. PHASE 2A
12. PHASE 2B

Down

1. POTENCY
3. ABNORMALITY
5. DATA DICTIONARY
7. CSR
8. HUMANS
11. ADR

CSR: Clinical Study Report; **ADR**: Adverse Drug Reactions

Crossword # 63

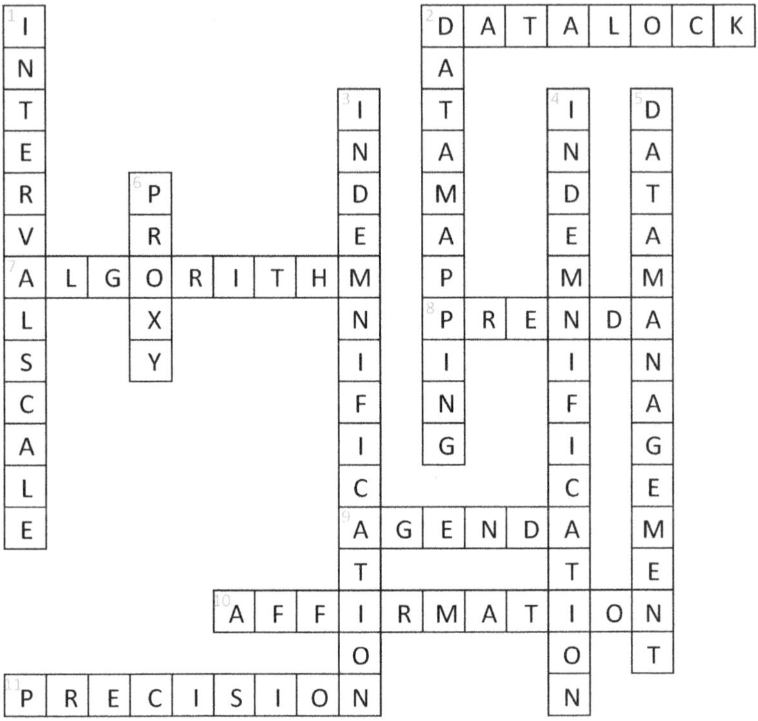

Across

2. DATA LOCK
7. ALGORITHM
8. PRE NDA
9. AGENDA
10. AFFIRMATION
11. PRECISION

Down

1. INTERVAL SCALE
2. DATA MAPPING
3. INDEMNIFICATION
4. INDEMNIFICATION
5. DATA MANAGEMENT
6. PROXY

Crossword # 64

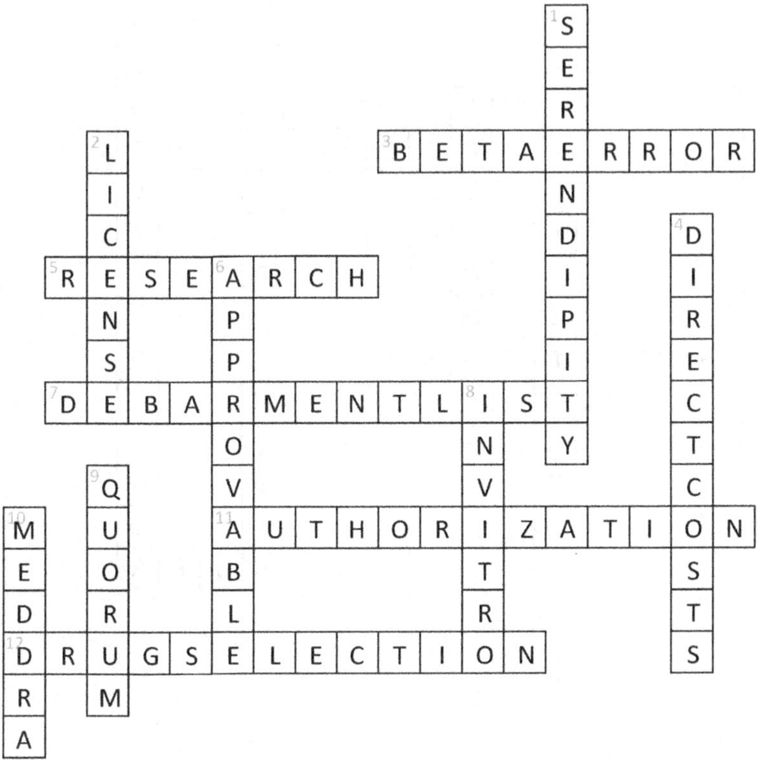

Across

3. BETA ERROR
5. RESEARCH
7. DEBARMENT LIST
11. AUTHORIZATION
12. DRUG SELECTION

Down

1. SERENDIPITY
2. LICENSE
4. DIRECT COSTS
6. APPROVABLE
8. IN VITRO
9. QUORUM
10. MedDRA

MedDRA: Medical Dictionary for Regulatory Activities

Crossword # 65

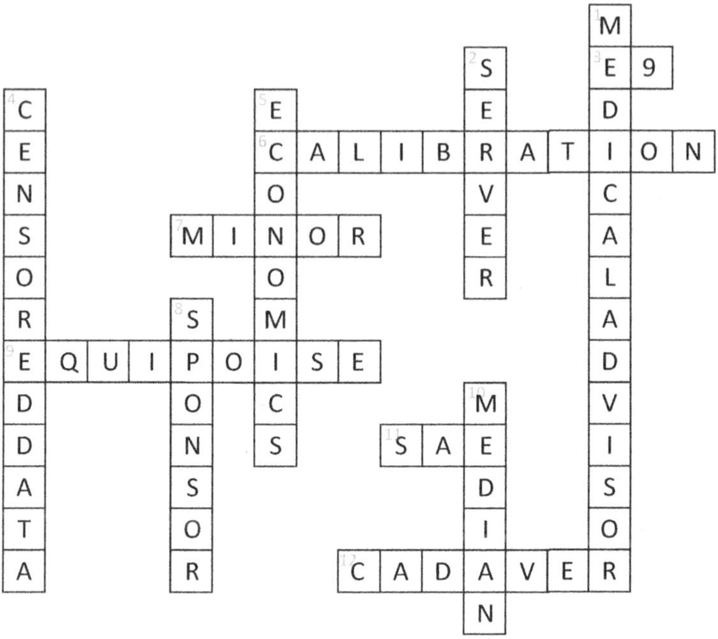

Across

3. E9
6. CALIBRATION
7. MINOR
9. EQUIPOISE
11. SAE
12. CADAVER

Down

1. MEDICAL ADVISOR
2. SERVER
4. CENSORED DATA
5. ECONOMICS
8. SPONSOR
10. MEDIAN

SAE: Serious Adverse Event

Crossword # 66

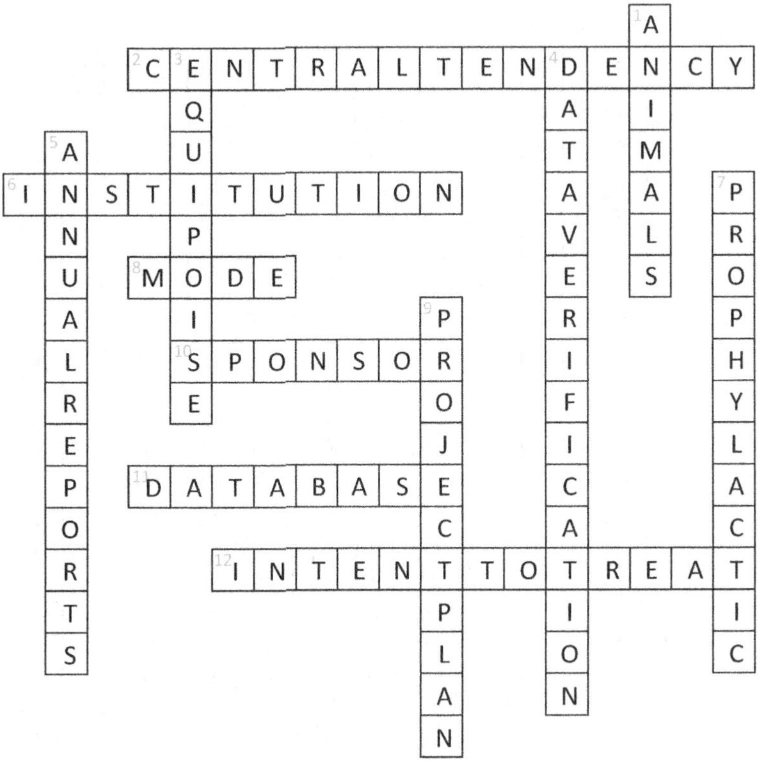

Across

2. CENTRAL TENDENCY
6. INSTITUTION
8. MODE
10. SPONSOR
11. DATABASE
12. INTENT TO TREAT

Down

1. ANIMALS
3. EQUIPOISE
4. DATA VERIFICATION
5. ANNUAL REPORTS
7. PROPHYLACTIC
9. PROJECT PLAN

Crossword # 67

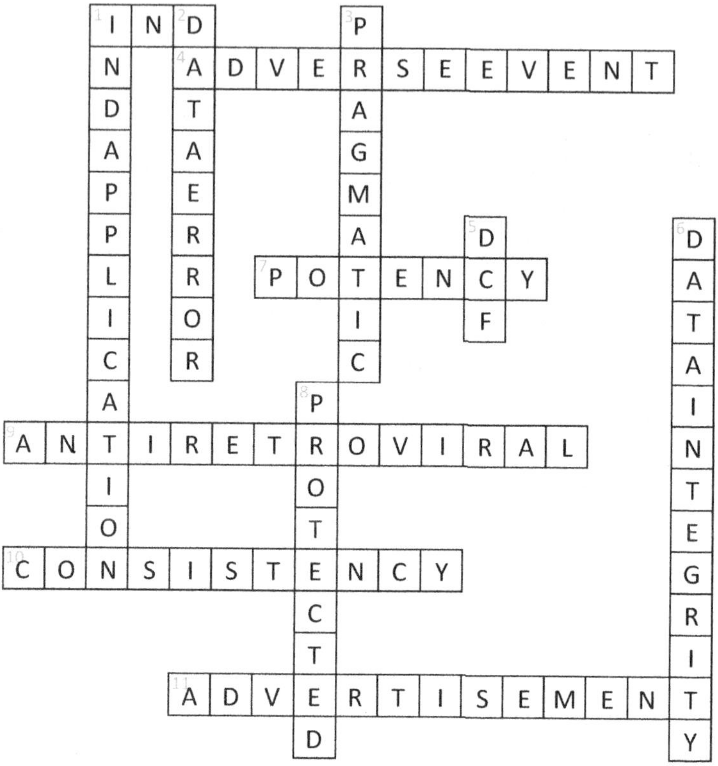

Across

1. IND
4. ADVERSE EVENT
7. POTENCY
9. ANTIRETROVIRAL
10. CONSISTENCY
11. ADVERTISEMENT

Down

1. IND APPLICATION
2. DATA ERROR
3. PRAGMATIC
5. DCF
6. DATA INTEGRITY
8. PROTECTED

IND: Investigational New Drug; **DCF**: Data Clarification Form

Crossword # 68

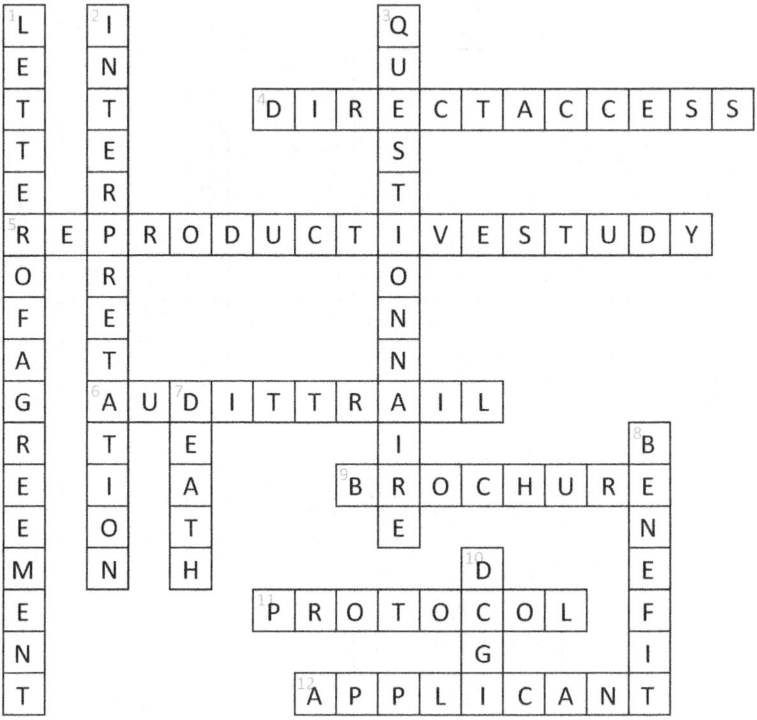

Across

4. DIRECT ACCESS
5. REPRODUCTIVE STUDY
6. AUDIT TRAIL
9. BROCHURE
11. PROTOCOL
12. APPLICANT

Down

1. LETTER OF AGREEMENT
2. INTERPRETATION
3. QUESTIONNAIRE
7. DEATH
8. BENEFIT
10. DCGI

DCGI: Drug Controller General of India

Crossword # 69

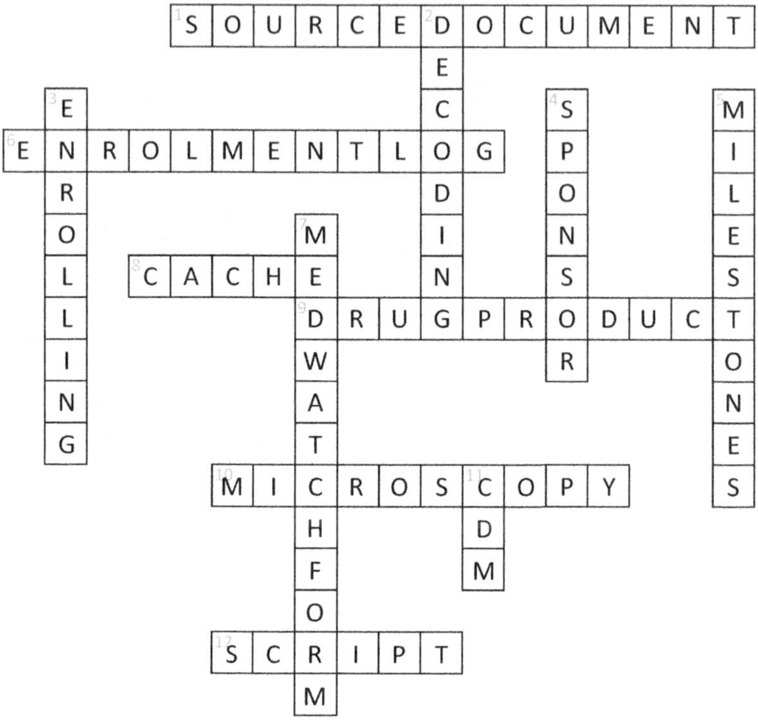

Across

1. SOURCE DOCUMENT
6. ENROLMENT LOG
8. CACHE
9. DRUG PRODUCT
10. MICROSCOPY
12. SCRIPT

Down

2. DECODING
3. ENROLLING
4. SPONSOR
5. MILESTONES
7. MEDWATCH FORM
11. CDM

CDM: Clinical Data Manager

Crossword # 70

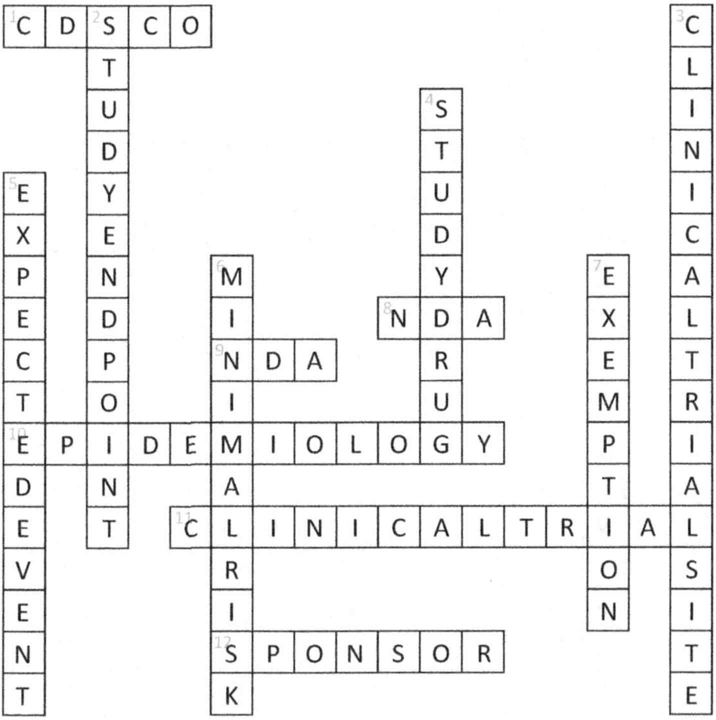

Across

1. CDSCO
8. NDA
9. NDA
10. EPIDEMIOLOGY
11. CLINICAL TRIAL
12. SPONSOR

Down

2. STUDY ENDPOINT
3. CLINICAL TRIAL SITE
4. STUDY DRUG
5. EXPECTED EVENT
6. MINIMAL RISK
7. EXEMPTION

CDSCO: Central Drug Standard Control Organization; **NDA**: Non Disclosure Agreement; **NDA**: New Drug Application

Crossword # 71

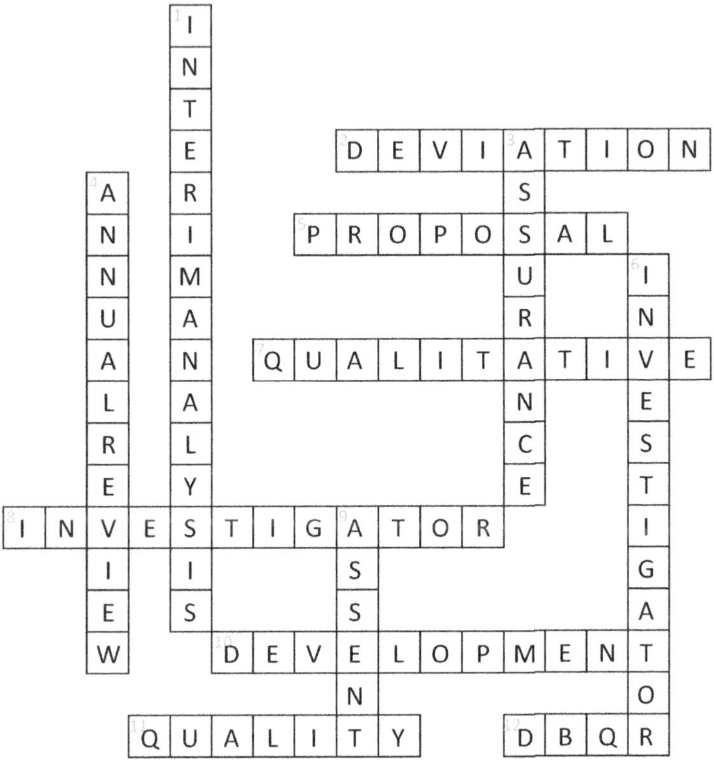

Across

2. DEVIATION
5. PROPOSAL
7. QUALITATIVE
8. INVESTIGATOR
10. DEVELOPMENT
11. QUALITY
12. DBQR

Down

1. INTERIM ANALYSIS
3. ASSURANCE
4. ANNUAL REVIEW
6. INVESTIGATOR
9. ASSENT

DBQR: Database Quality Review

Crossword # 72

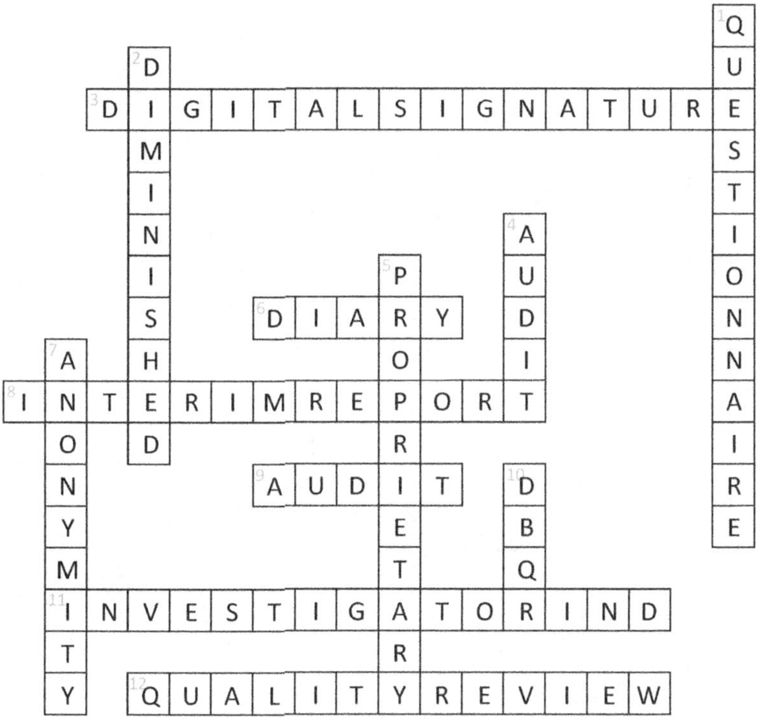

Across

3. DIGITAL SIGNATURE
6. DIARY
8. INTERIM REPORT
9. AUDIT
11. INVESTIGATOR IND
12. QUALITY REVIEW

Down

1. QUESTIONNAIRE
2. DIMINISHED
4. AUDIT
5. PROPRIETARY
7. ANONYMITY
10. DBQR

DBQR: Database Quality Review

Crossword # 73

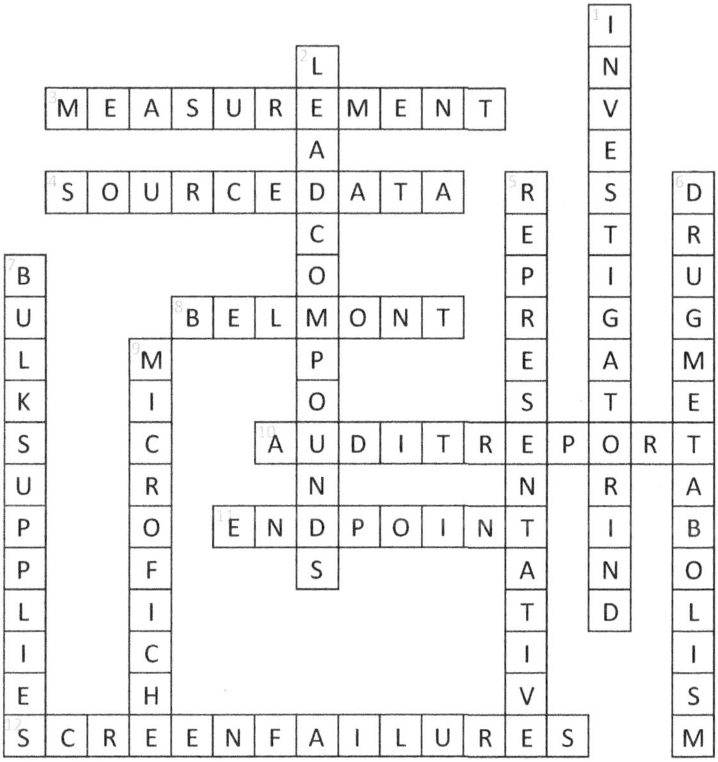

Across

3. MEASUREMENT
4. SOURCE DATA
8. BELMONT
10. AUDIT REPORT
11. ENDPOINT
12. SCREEN FAILURES

Down

1. INVESTIGATOR IND
2. LEAD COMPOUNDS
5. REPRESENTATIVE
6. DRUG METABOLISM
7. BULK SUPPLIES
9. MICROFICHE

Crossword # 74

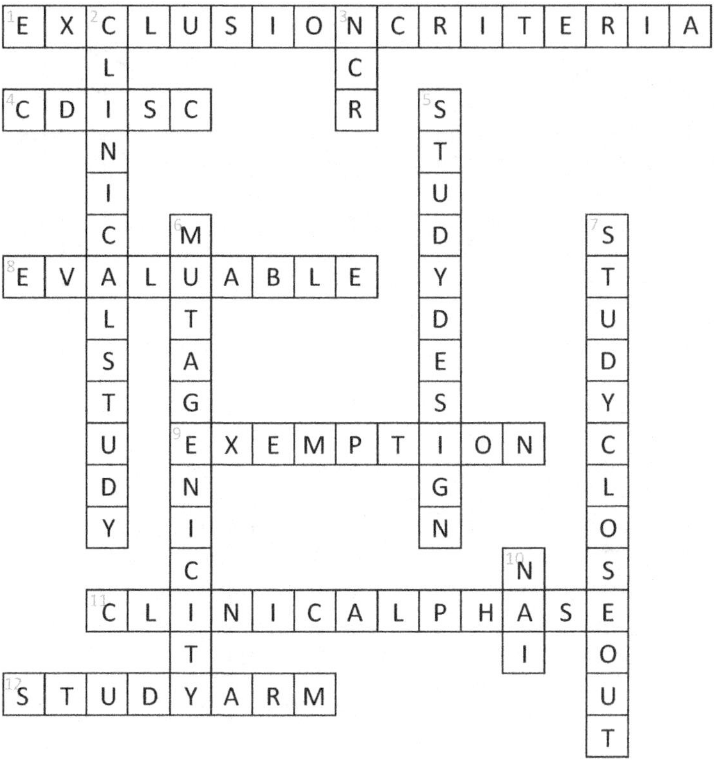

Across

1. EXCLUSION CRITERIA
4. CDISC
8. EVALUABLE
9. EXEMPTION
11. CLINICAL PHASE
12. STUDY ARM

Down

2. CLINICAL STUDY
3. NCR
5. STUDY DESIGN
6. MUTAGENICITY
7. STUDY CLOSEOUT
10. NAI

CDISC: Clinical Data Interchange Standards Consortium; **NCR**: No Carbon Required; **NAI**: No Action Indicated

Crossword # 75

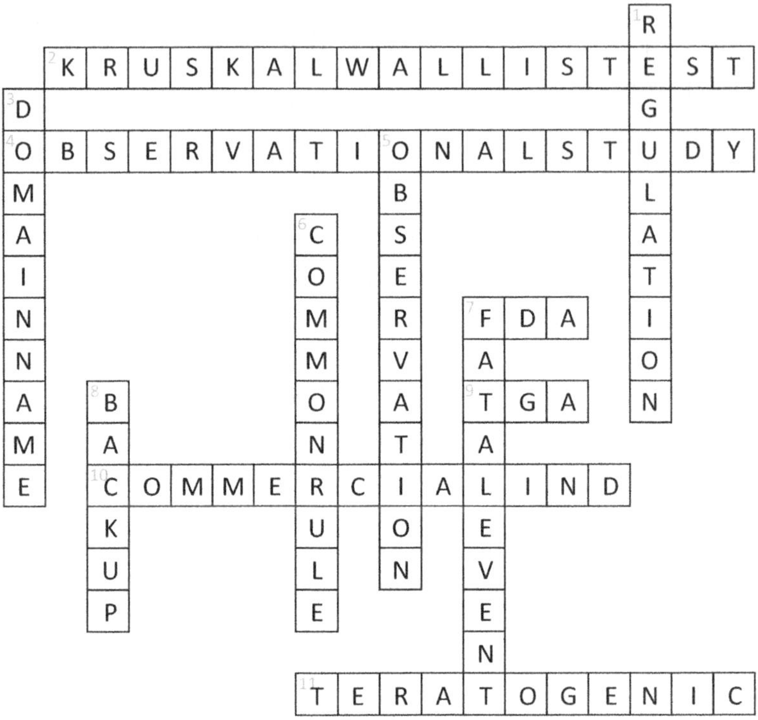

Across

2. KRUSKAL WALLIS TEST
4. OBSERVATIONAL STUDY
7. FDA
9. TGA
10. COMMERCIAL IND
11. TERATOGENIC

Down

1. REGULATION
3. DOMAIN NAME
5. OBSERVATION
6. COMMON RULE
7. FATAL EVENT
8. BACKUP

FDA: Food and Drug Administration; **TGA**: Therapeutics Goods Administration

Crossword # 76

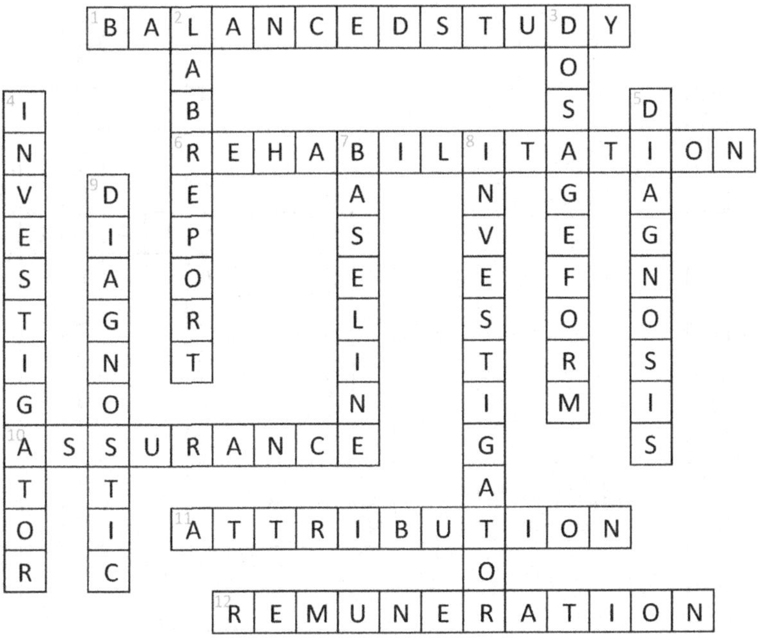

Across

1. BALANCED STUDY
6. REHABILITATION
10. ASSURANCE
11. ATTRIBUTION
12. REMUNERATION

Down

2. LAB REPORT
3. DOSAGE FORM
4. INVESTIGATOR
5. DIAGNOSIS
7. BASELINE
8. INVESTIGATOR
9. DIAGNOSTIC

Crossword # 77

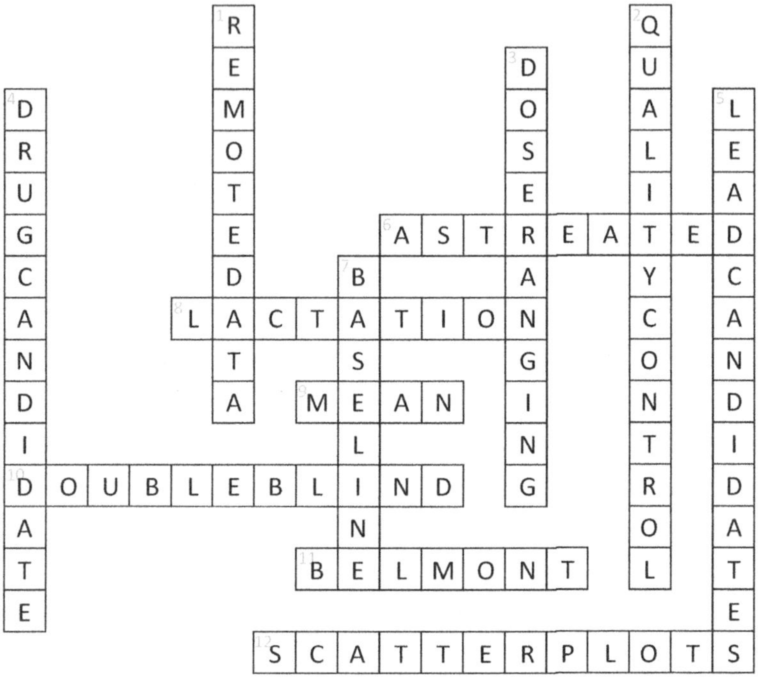

Across

6. AS TREATED
8. LACTATION
9. MEAN
10. DOUBLE BLIND
11. BELMONT
12. SCATTER PLOTS

Down

1. REMOTE DATA
2. QUALITY CONTROL
3. DOSE RANGING
4. DRUG CANDIDATE
5. LEAD CANDIDATES
7. BASELINE

Crossword # 78

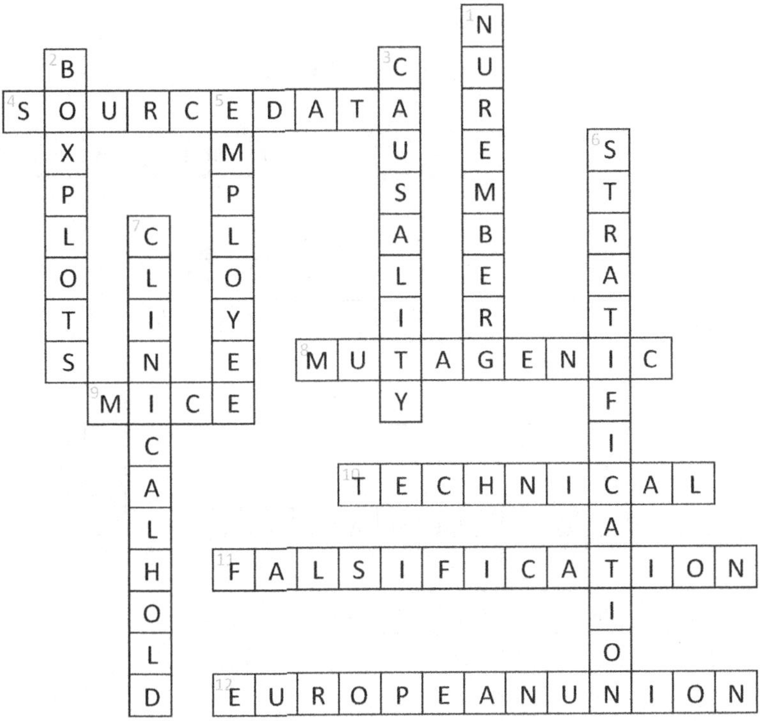

Across

4. SOURCE DATA
8. MUTAGENIC
9. MICE
10. TECHNICAL
11. FALSIFICATION
12. EUROPEAN UNION

Down

1. NUREMBERG
2. BOX PLOTS
3. CAUSALITY
5. EMPLOYEE
6. STRATIFICATION
7. CLINICAL HOLD

Crossword # 79

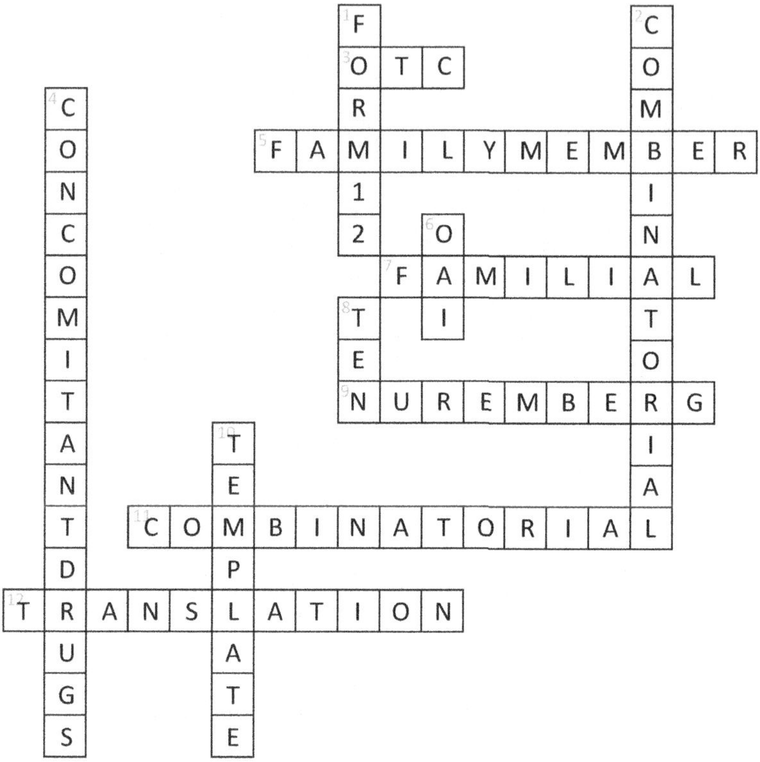

Across

3. OTC
5. FAMILY MEMBER
7. FAMILIAL
9. NUREMBERG
11. COMBINATORIAL
12. TRANSLATION

Down

1. FORM 12
2. COMBINATORIAL
4. CONCOMITANT DRUGS
6. OAI
8. TEN
10. TEMPLATE

OTC: Over The Counter; **OAI**: Official Action Indicated

Crossword # 80

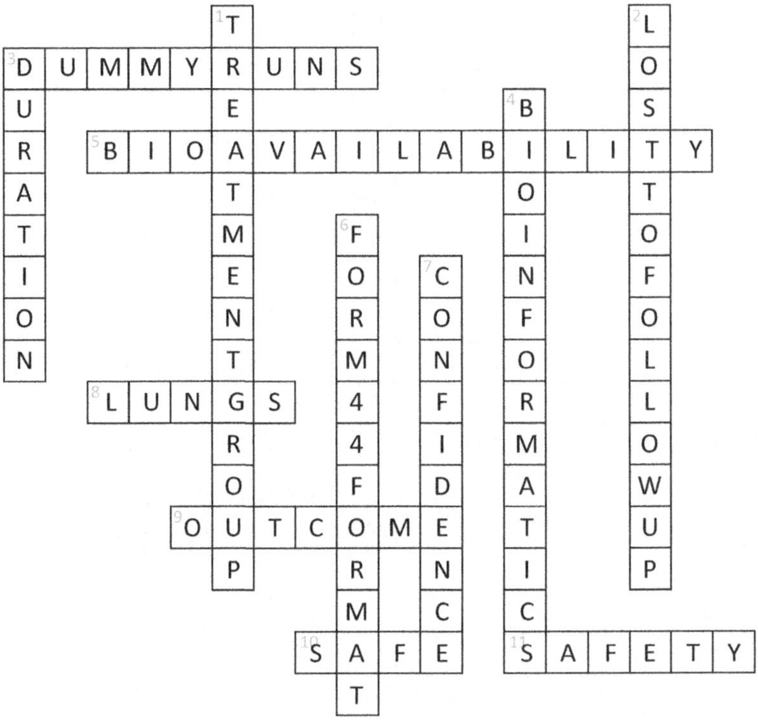

Across

3. DUMMY RUNS
5. BIOAVAILABILITY
8. LUNGS
9. OUTCOME
10. SAFE
11. SAFETY

Down

1. TREATMENT GROUP
2. LOST TO FOLLOW UP
3. DURATION
4. BIOINFORMATICS
6. FORM 44 FORMAT
7. CONFIDENCE

Crossword # 81

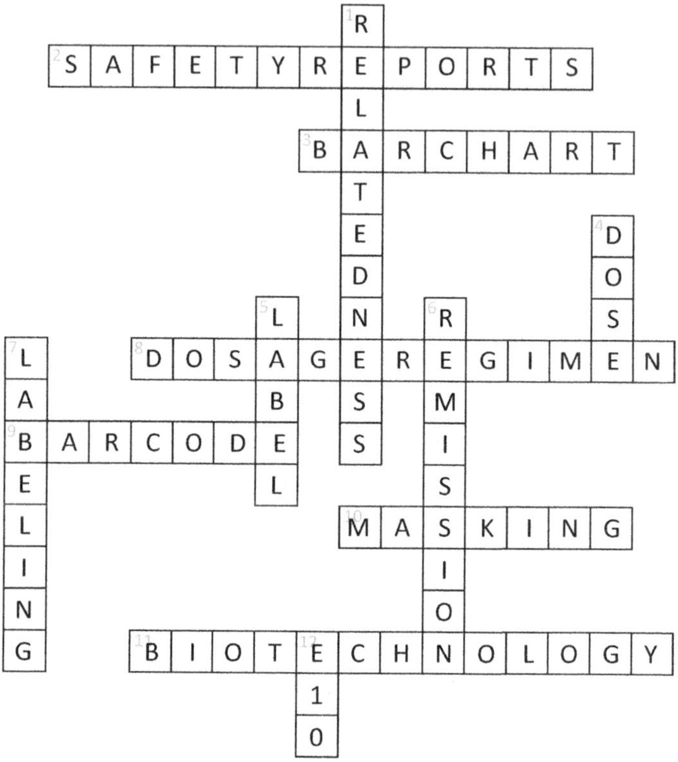

Across

2. SAFETY REPORTS
3. BAR CHART
8. DOSAGE REGIMEN
9. BARCODE
10. MASKING
11. BIOTECHNOLOGY

Down

1. RELATEDNESS
4. DOSE
5. LABEL
6. REMISSION
7. LABELING
12. E10

Crossword # 82

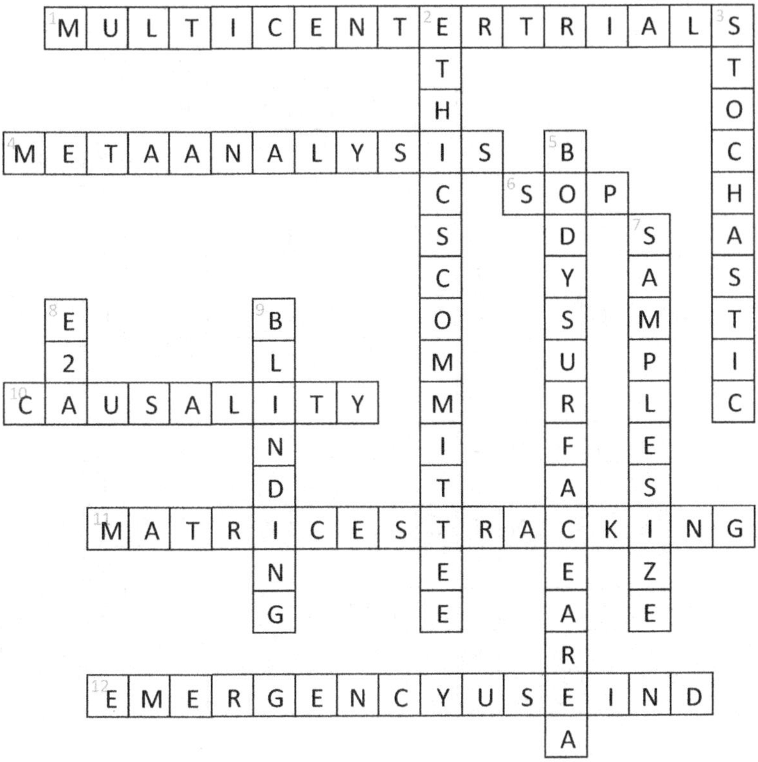

Across

1. MULTICENTER TRIALS
4. META ANALYSIS
6. SOP
10. CAUSALITY
11. MATRICES TRACKING
12. EMERGENCY USE IND

Down

2. ETHICS COMMITTEE
3. STOCHASTIC
5. BODY SURFACE AREA
7. SAMPLE SIZE
8. E2A
9. BLINDING

SOP: Standard Operating Procedure

Crossword # 83

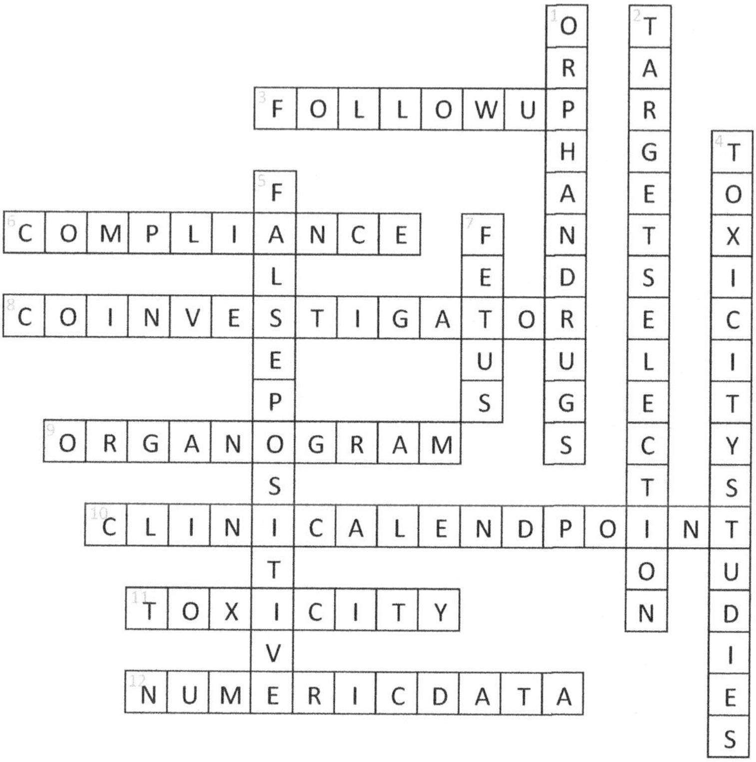

Across

3. FOLLOW UP
6. COMPLIANCE
8. CO INVESTIGATOR
9. ORGANOGRAM
10. CLINICAL ENDPOINT
11. TOXICITY
12. NUMERIC DATA

Down

1. ORPHAN DRUGS
2. TARGET SELECTION
4. TOXICITY STUDIES
5. FALSE POSITIVE
7. FETUS

Crossword # 84

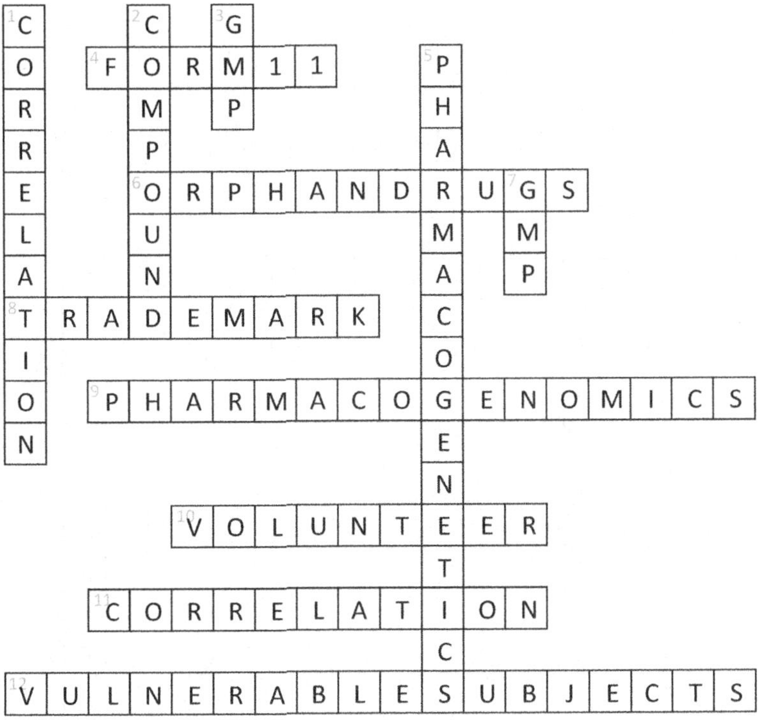

Across

4. FORM 11
6. ORPHAN DRUGS
8. TRADEMARK
9. PHARMACOGENOMICS
10. VOLUNTEER
11. CORRELATION
12. VULNERABLE SUBJECTS

Down

1. CORRELATION
2. COMPOUND
3. GMP
5. PHARMACOGENETICS
7. GMP

GMP: Good Manufacturing Practice

Crossword # 85

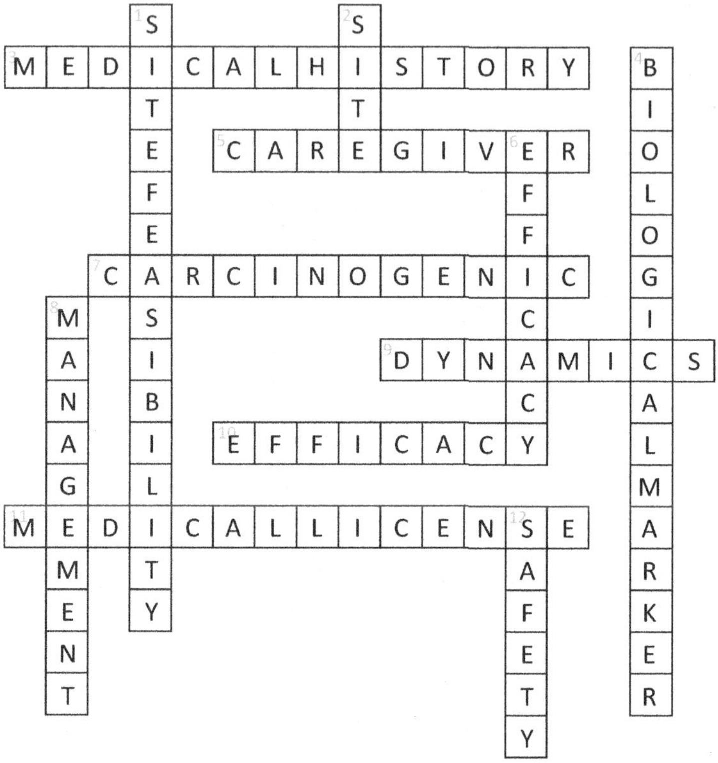

Across

3. MEDICAL HISTORY
5. CAREGIVER
7. CARCINOGENIC
9. DYNAMICS
10. EFFICACY
11. MEDICAL LICENSE

Down

1. SITE FEASIBILITY
2. SITE
4. BIOLOGICAL MARKER
6. EFFICACY
8. MANAGEMENT
12. SAFETY

Crossword # 86

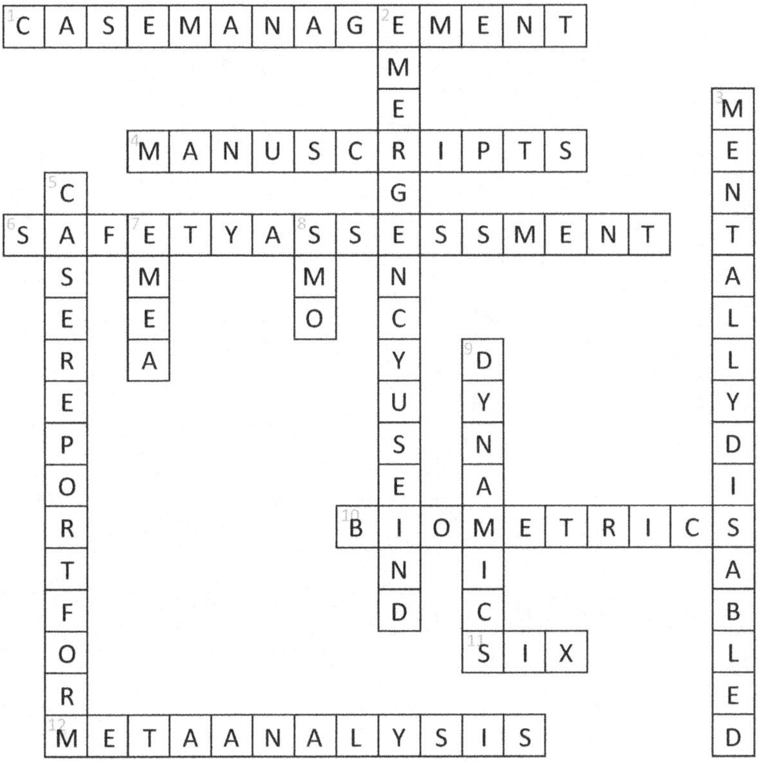

Across

1. CASE MANAGEMENT
4. MANUSCRIPTS
6. SAFETY ASSESSMENT
10. BIOMETRICS
11. SIX
12. META ANALYSIS

Down

2. EMERGENCY USE IND
3. MENTALLY DISABLED
5. CASE REPORT FORM
7. EMEA
8. SMO
9. DYNAMICS

EMEA: European Agency for the Evaluation of Medicinal Products; **SMO**: Site Management Organization

Crossword # 87

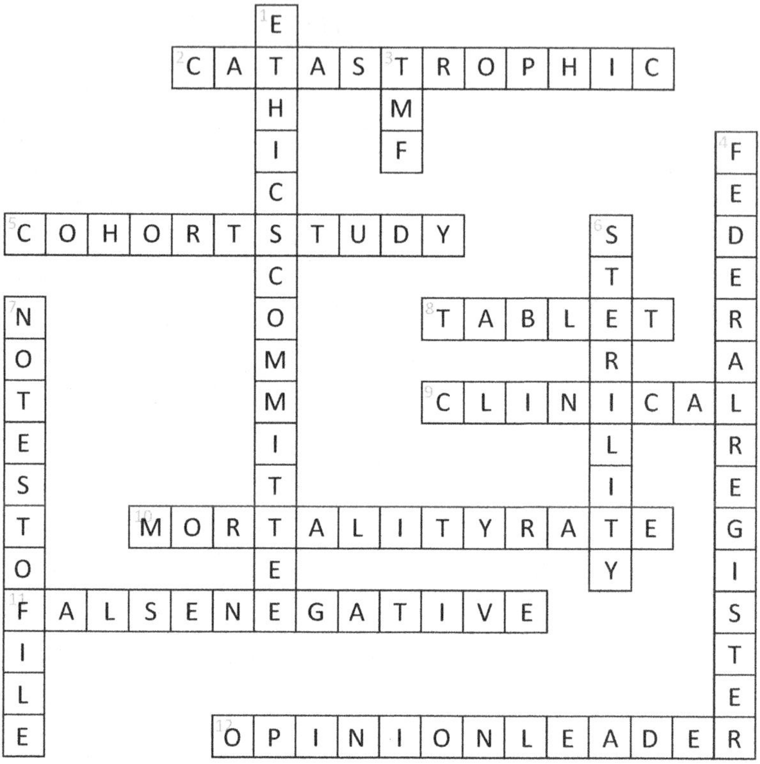

Across

2. CATASTROPHIC
5. COHORT STUDY
8. TABLET
9. CLINICAL
10. MORTALITY RATE
11. FALSE NEGATIVE
12. OPINION LEADER

Down

1. ETHICS COMMITTEE
3. TMF
4. FEDERAL REGISTER
6. STERILITY
7. NOTES TO FILE

TMF: Trial Master File

Crossword # 88

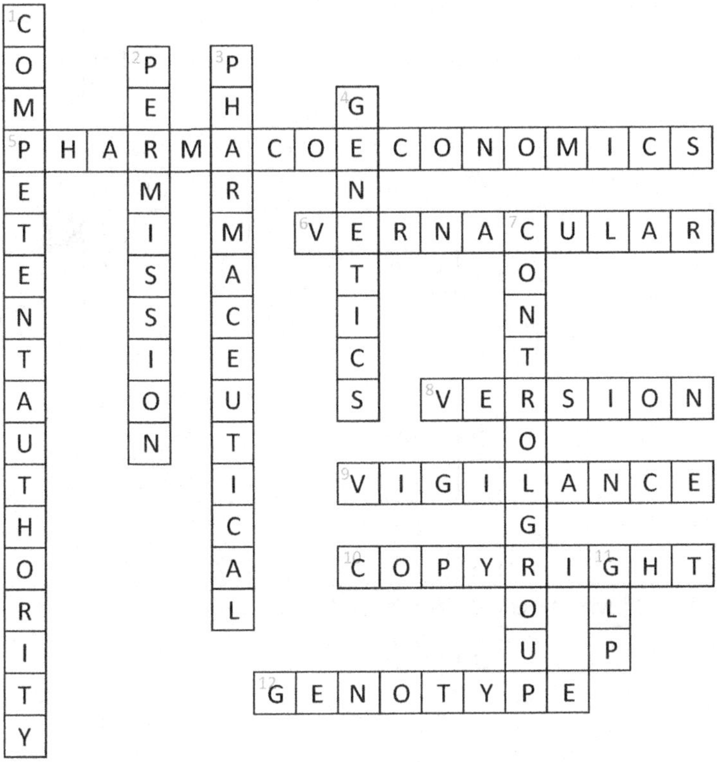

Across

5. PHARMACOECONOMICS
6. VERNACULAR
8. VERSION
9. VIGILANCE
10. COPYRIGHT
12. GENOTYPE

Down

1. COMPETENT AUTHORITY
2. PERMISSION
3. PHARMACEUTICAL
4. GENETICS
7. CONTROL GROUP
11. GLP

GLP: Good Laboratory Practices

Crossword # 89

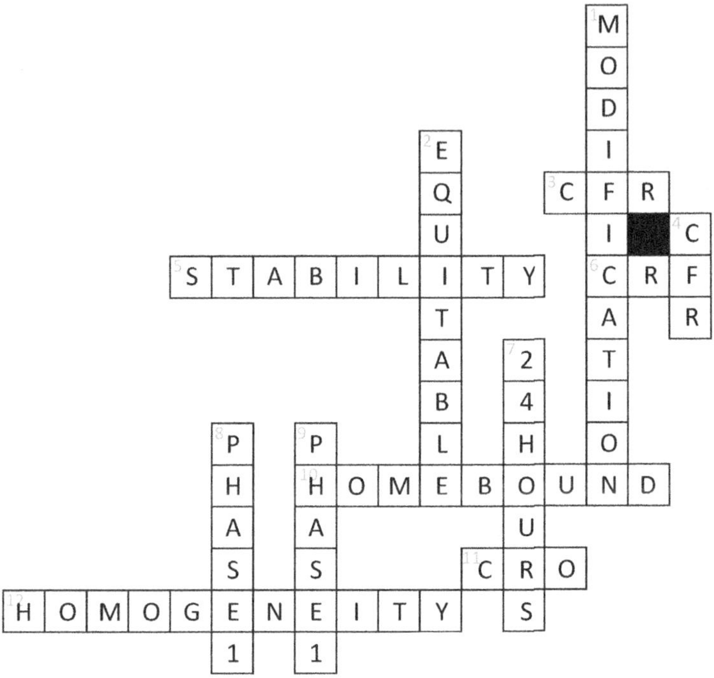

Across

3. CFR
5. STABILITY
6. CRF
10. HOME BOUND
11. CRO
12. HOMOGENEITY

Down

1. MODIFICATION
2. EQUITABLE
4. CFR
7. 24 HOURS
8. PHASE 1
9. PHASE 1

CRF: Case Report Form; **CRO**: Contract Research Organization; **CFR**: Code of Federal Regulation

Crossword # 90

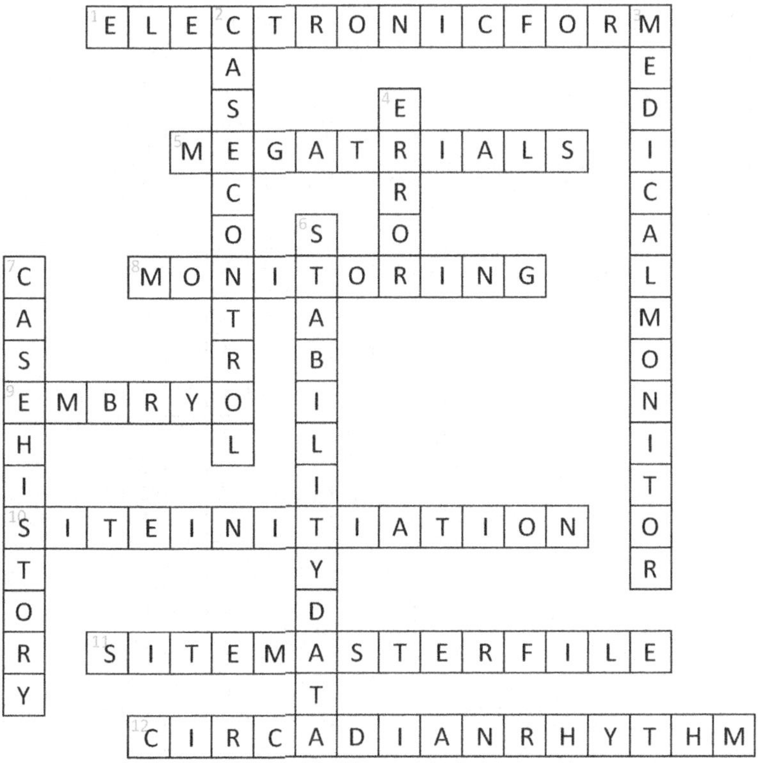

Across

1. ELECTRONIC FORM
5. MEGA TRIALS
8. MONITORING
9. EMBRYO
10. SITE INITIATION
11. SITE MASTER FILE
12. CIRCADIAN RHYTHM

Down

2. CASE CONTROL
3. MEDICAL MONITOR
4. ERROR
6. STABILITY DATA
7. CASE HISTORY

Crossword # 91

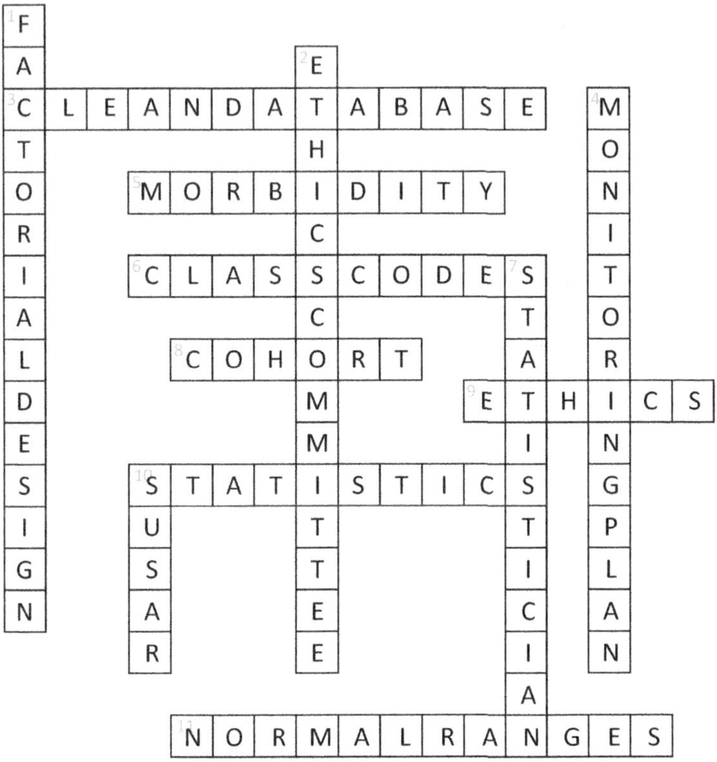

Across

3. CLEAN DATABASE
5. MORBIDITY
6. CLASS CODES
8. COHORT
9. ETHICS
10. STATISTICS
11. NORMAL RANGES

Down

1. FACTORIAL DESIGN
2. ETHICS COMMITTEE
4. MONITORING PLAN
7. STATISTICIAN
10. SUSAR

Crossword # 92

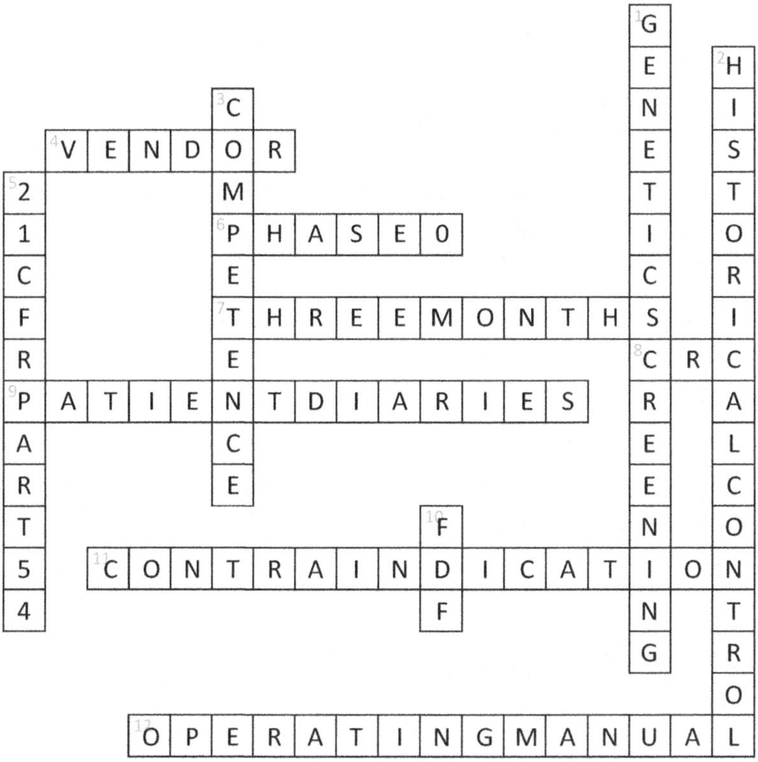

Across

4. VENDOR
6. PHASE 0
7. THREE MONTHS
8. CRC
9. PATIENT DIARIES
11. CONTRAINDICATION
12. OPERATING MANUAL

Down

1. GENETIC SCREENING
2. HISTORICAL CONTROL
3. COMPETENCE
5. 21 CFR PART 54
10. FDF

CRC : Clinical Research Coordinator; **FDF** : Financial Disclosure Form

Crossword # 93

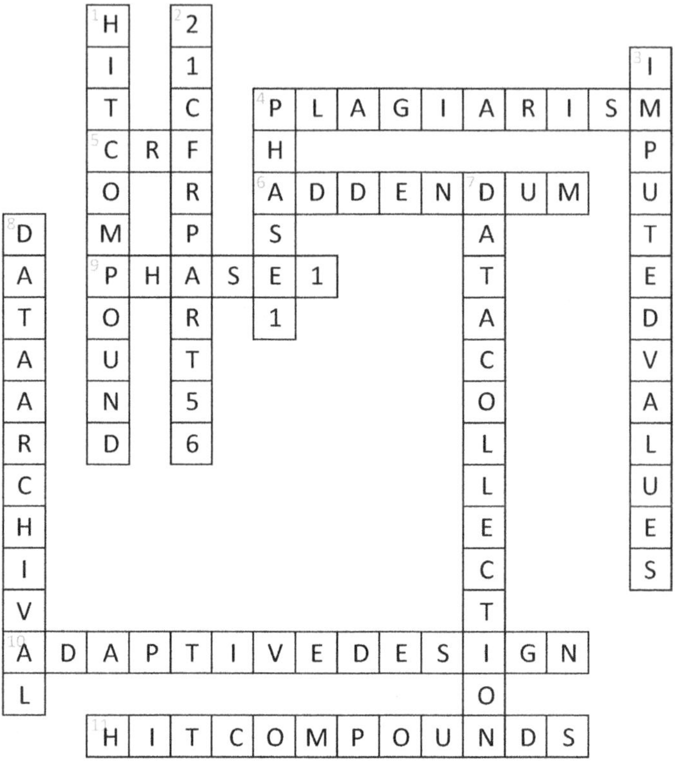

Across

4. PLAGIARISM
5. CRF
6. ADDENDUM
9. PHASE 1
10. ADAPTIVE DESIGN
11. HIT COMPOUNDS

Down

1. HIT COMPOUND
2. 21 CFR PART 56
3. IMPUTED VALUES
4. PHASE 1
7. DATA COLLECTION
8. DATA ARCHIVAL

CRF: Case Report Form

Crossword # 94

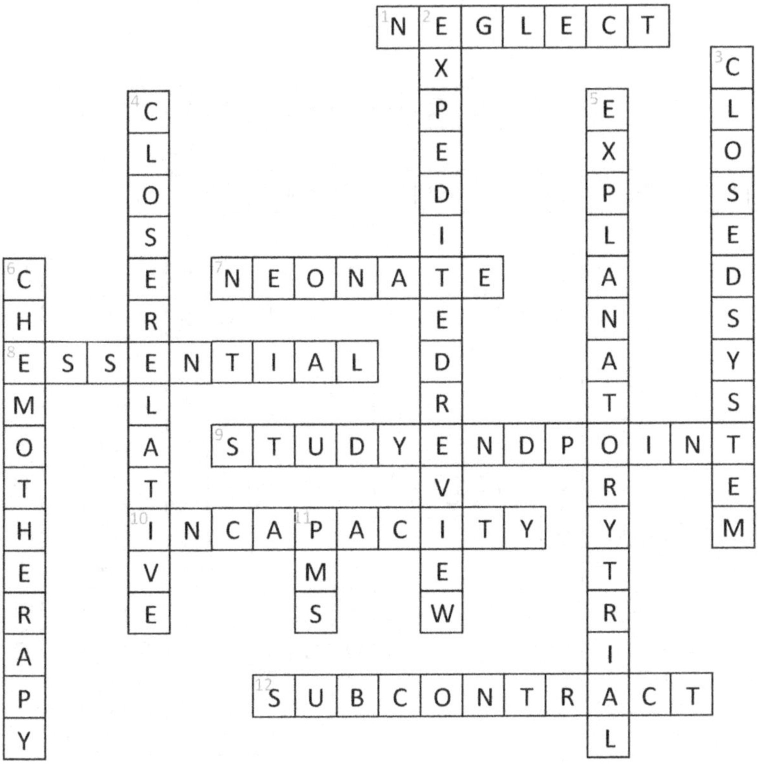

Across

1. NEGLECT
7. NEONATE
8. ESSENTIAL
9. STUDY ENDPOINT
10. INCAPACITY
12. SUB CONTRACT

Down

2. EXPEDITED REVIEW
3. CLOSED SYSTEM
4. CLOSE RELATIVE
5. EXPLANATORY TRIAL
6. CHEMOTHERAPY
11. PMS

PMS: Post Marketing Surveillance

Crossword # 95

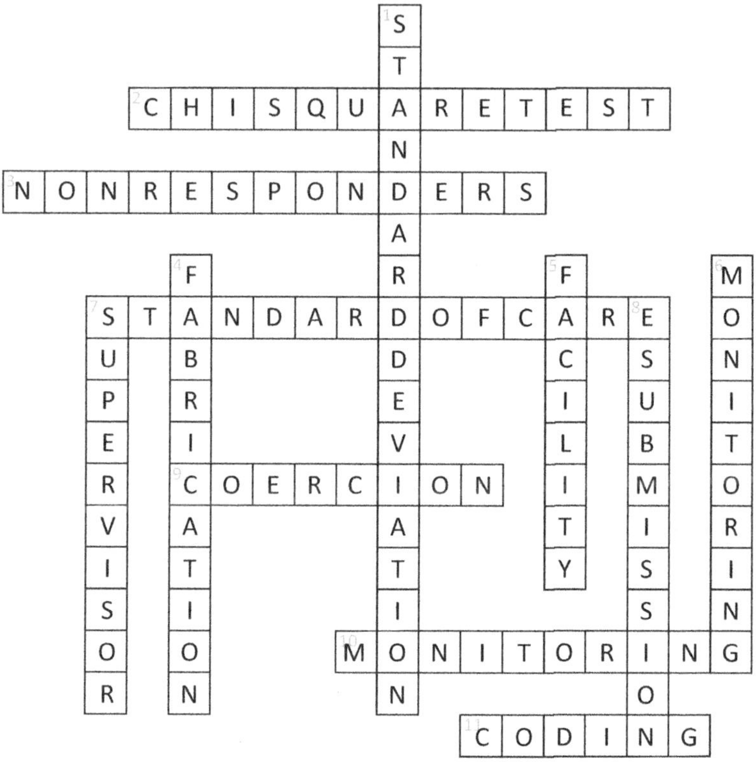

Across

2. CHI SQUARE TEST
3. NON RESPONDERS
7. STANDARD OF CARE
9. COERCION
10. MONITORING
11. CODING

Down

1. STANDARD DEVIATION
4. FABRICATION
5. FACILITY
6. MONITORING
7. SUPERVISOR
8. e SUBMISSION

Crossword # 96

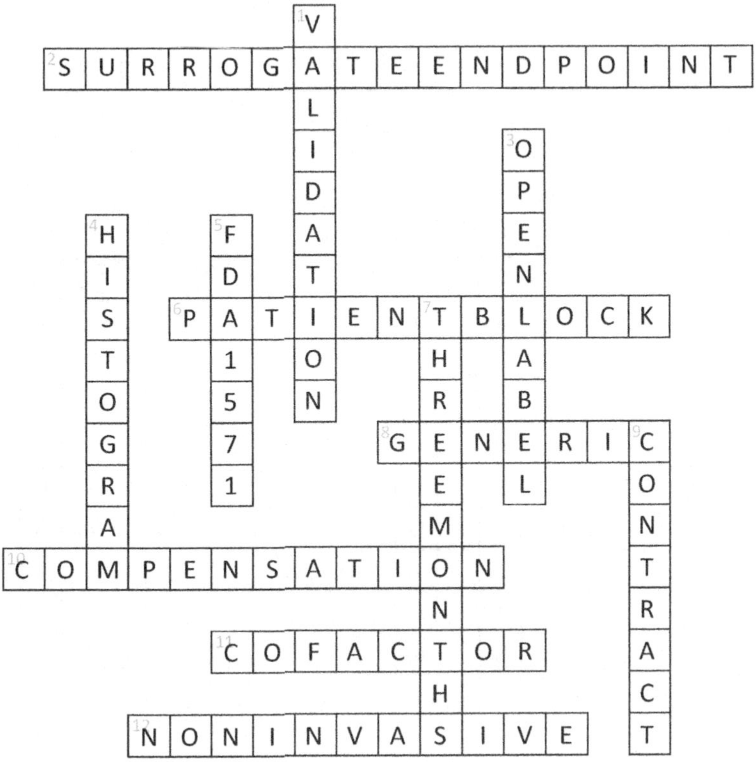

Across

2. SURROGATE ENDPOINT
6. PATIENT BLOCK
8. GENERIC
10. COMPENSATION
11. COFACTOR
12. NON INVASIVE

Down

1. VALIDATION
3. OPEN LABEL
4. HISTOGRAM
5. FDA 1571
7. THREE MONTHS
9. CONTRACT

Crossword # 97

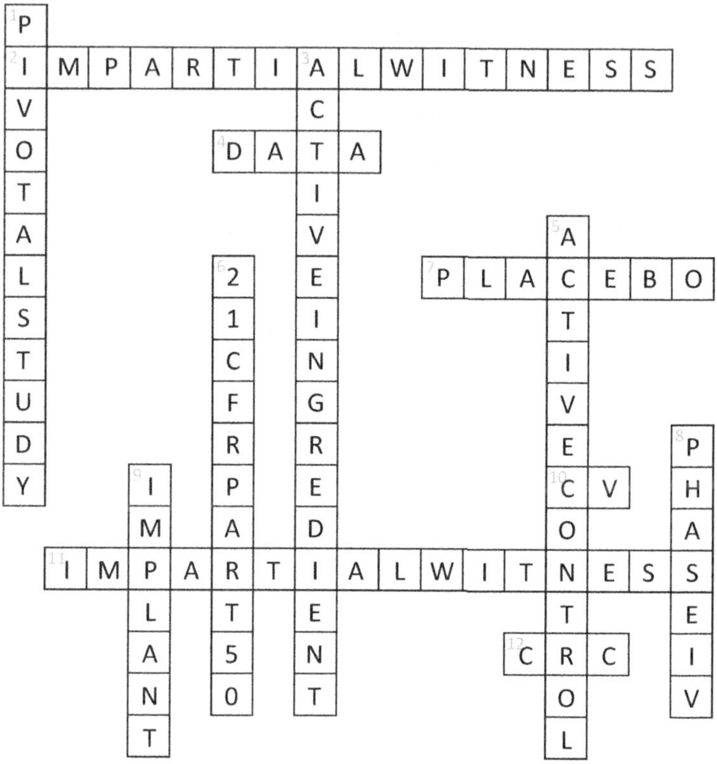

Across

2. IMPARTIAL WITNESS
4. DATA
7. PLACEBO
10. CV
11. IMPARTIAL WITNESS
12. CRC

Down

1. PIVOTAL STUDY
3. ACTIVE INGREDIENT
5. ACTIVE CONTROL
6. 21 CFR PART 50
8. PHASE IV
9. IMPLANT

CV: Curriculum Vitae; **CRC**: Clinical Research Coordinator

Crossword # 98

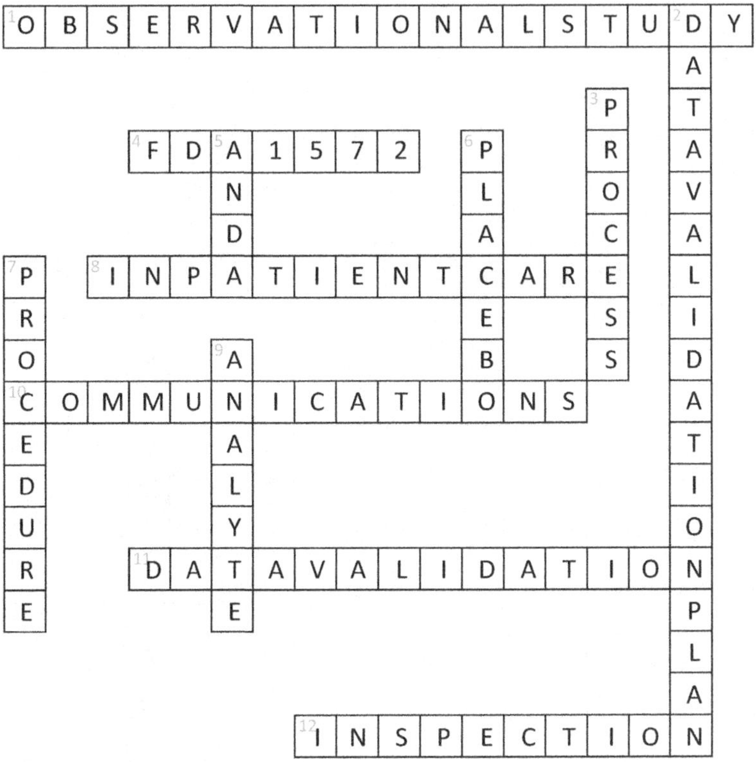

Across

1. OBSERVATIONAL STUDY
4. FDA 1572
8. INPATIENT CARE
10. COMMUNICATIONS
11. DATA VALIDATION
12. INSPECTION

Down

2. DATA VALIDATION PLAN
3. PROCESS
5. ANDA
6. PLACEBO
7. PROCEDURE
9. ANALYTE

ANDA: Abbreviated New Drug Application

Crossword # 99

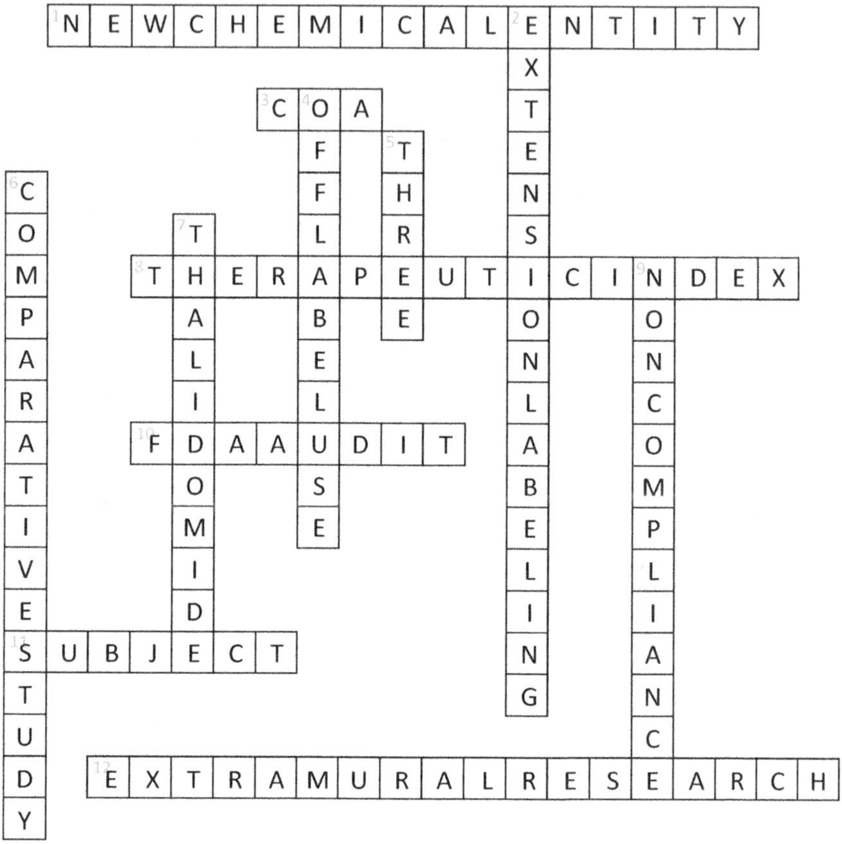

Across

1. NEW CHEMICAL ENTITY
3. COA
8. THERAPEUTIC INDEX
10. FDA AUDIT
11. SUBJECT
12. EXTRAMURAL RESEARCH

Down

2. EXTENSION LABELING
4. OFF LABEL USE
5. THREE
6. COMPARATIVE STUDY
7. THALIDOMIDE
9. NON COMPLIANCE

COA: Certificate of Analysis

Crossword # 100

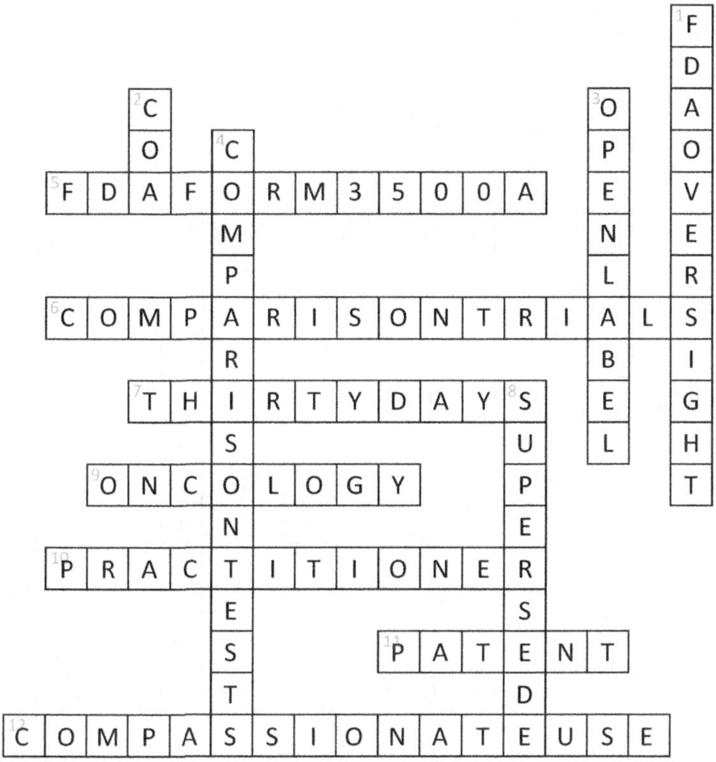

Across

5. FDA FORM 3500A
6. COMPARISON TRIALS
7. THIRTY DAYS
9. ONCOLOGY
10. PRACTITIONER
11. PATENT
12. COMPASSIONATE USE

Down

1. FDA OVERSIGHT
2. COA
3. OPEN LABEL
4. COMPARISON TESTS
8. SUPERSEDE

Crossword # 101

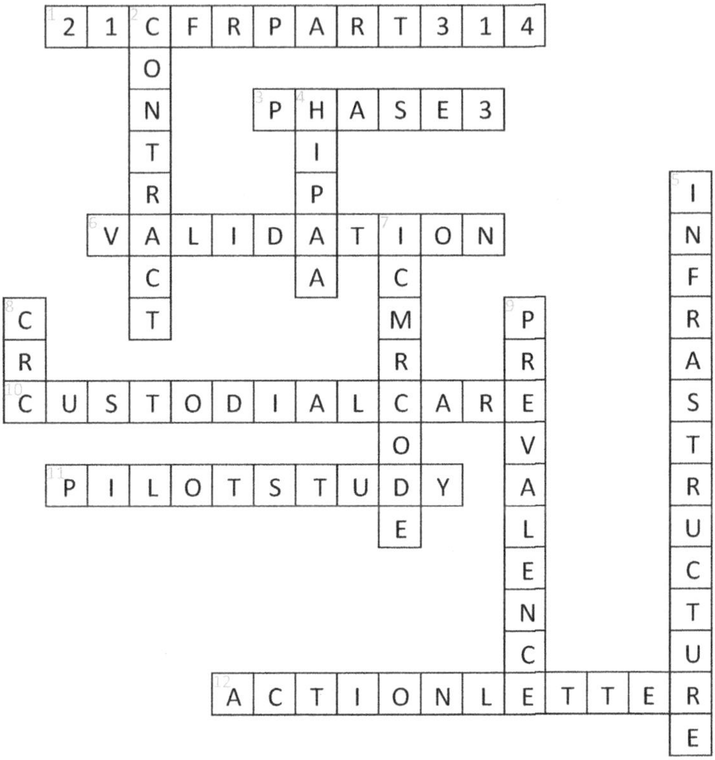

Across

1. 21 CFR PART 314
3. PHASE 3
6. VALIDATION
10. CUSTODIAL CARE
11. PILOT STUDY
12. ACTION LETTER

Down

2. CONTRACT
4. HIPAA
5. INFRASTRUCTURE
7. ICMR CODE
8. CRC
9. PREVALENCE

HIPAA: Health Insurance Portability and Accountability Act; **CRC**: Clinical Research Coordinator

Crossword # 102

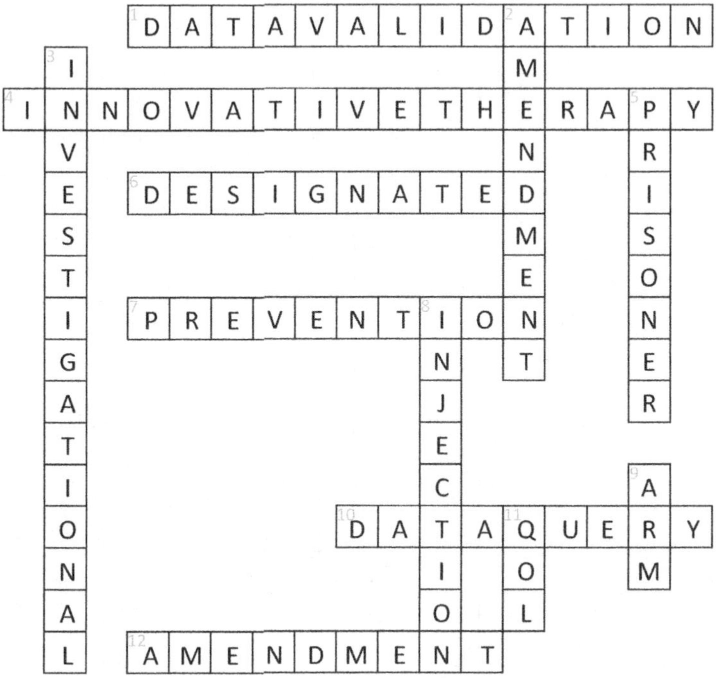

Across

1. DATA VALIDATION
4. INNOVATIVE THERAPY
6. DESIGNATED
7. PREVENTION
10. DATA QUERY
12. AMENDMENT

Down

2. AMENDMENT
3. INVESTIGATIONAL
5. PRISONER
8. INJECTION
9. ARM
11. QOL

QOL: Quality of Life

Crossword # 103

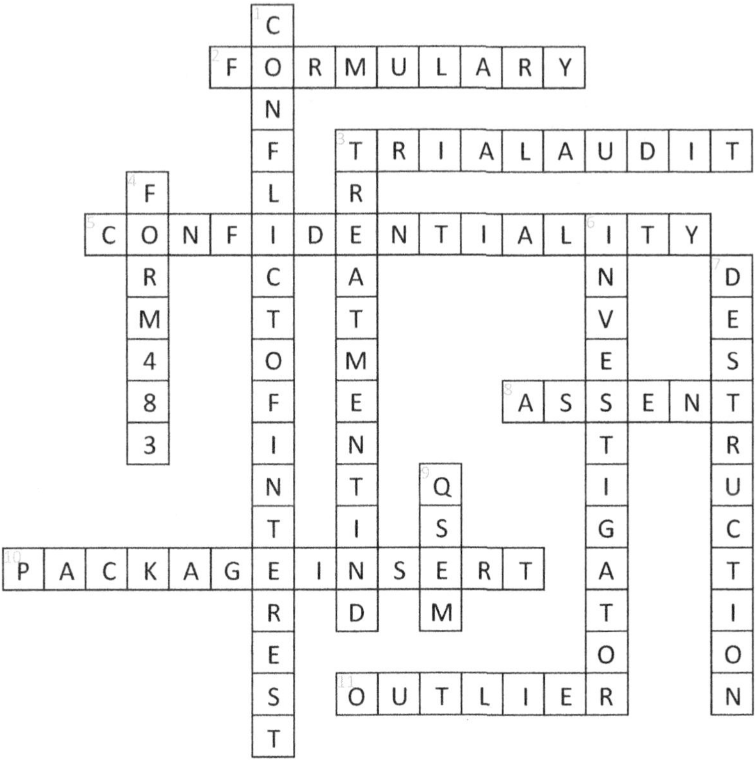

Across

2. FORMULARY
3. TRIAL AUDIT
5. CONFIDENTIALITY
8. ASSENT
10. PACKAGE INSERT
11. OUTLIER

Down

1. CONFLICT OF INTEREST
3. TREATMENT IND
4. FORM 483
6. INVESTIGATOR
7. DESTRUCTION
9. QSEM

QSEM: Quality, Safety, Efficacy, Multidisciplinary

Crossword # 104

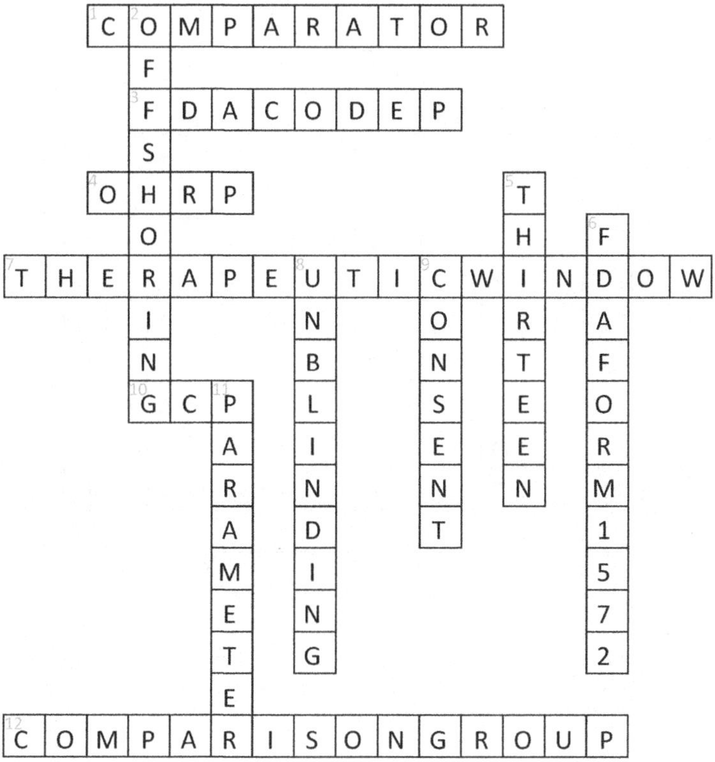

Across

1. COMPARATOR
3. FDA CODE P
4. OHRP
7. THERAPEUTIC WINDOW
10. GCP
12. COMPARISON GROUP

Down

2. OFF SHORING
5. THIRTEEN
6. FDA FORM 1572
8. UNBLINDING
9. CONSENT
11. PARAMETER

OHRP: Office for Human Research Protection; **GCP**: Good Clinical Practice

Crossword # 105

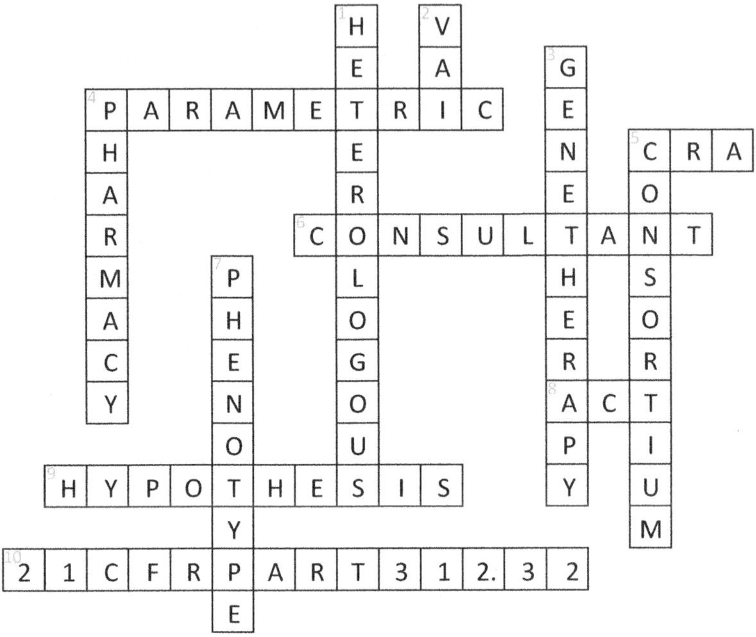

Across

4. PARAMETRIC
5. CRA
6. CONSULTANT
8. ACT
9. HYPOTHESIS
10. 21 CFR PART 312.32

Down

1. HETEROLOGOUS
2. VAI
3. GENE THERAPY
4. PHARMACY
5. CONSORTIUM
7. PHENOTYPE

CRA: Clinical Research Associate; **VAI**: Voluntary Action Indicated

Crossword # 106

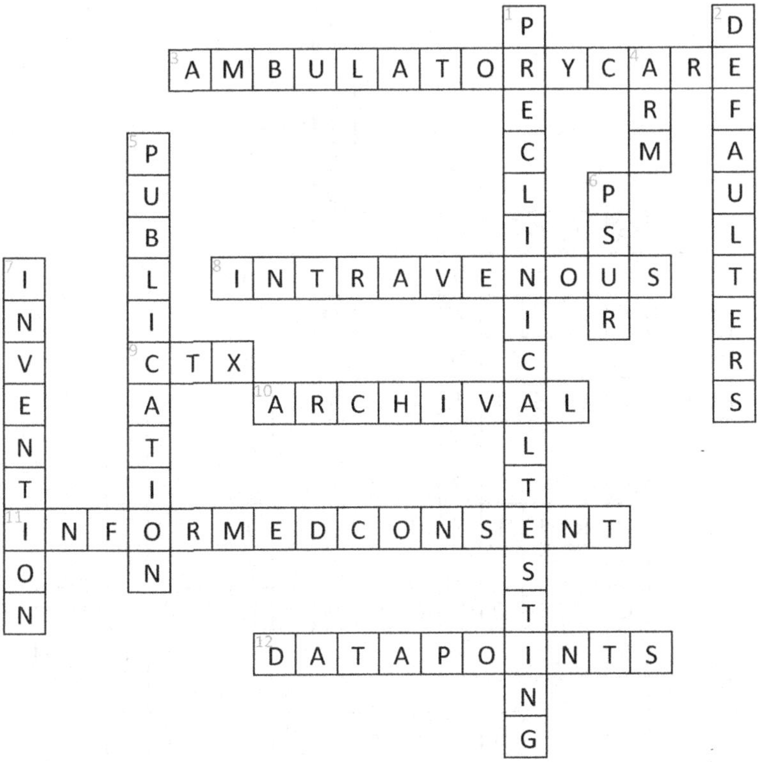

Across

3. AMBULATORY CARE
8. INTRAVENOUS
9. CTX
10. ARCHIVAL
11. INFORMED CONSENT
12. DATA POINTS

Down

1. PRE CLINICAL TESTING
2. DEFAULTERS
4. ARM
5. PUBLICATION
6. PSUR
7. INVENTION

PSUR: Periodic Safety Update Report

Crossword # 107

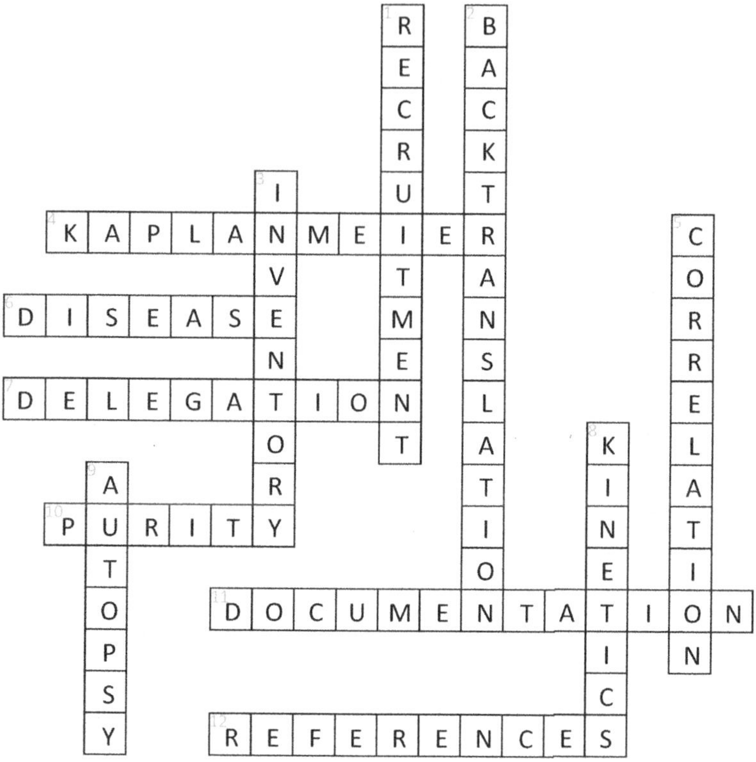

Across

4. KAPLAN MEIER
6. DISEASE
7. DELEGATION
10. PURITY
11. DOCUMENTATION
12. REFERENCES

Down

1. RECRUITMENT
2. BACK TRANSLATION
3. INVENTORY
5. CORRELATION
8. KINETICS
9. AUTOPSY

Crossword # 108

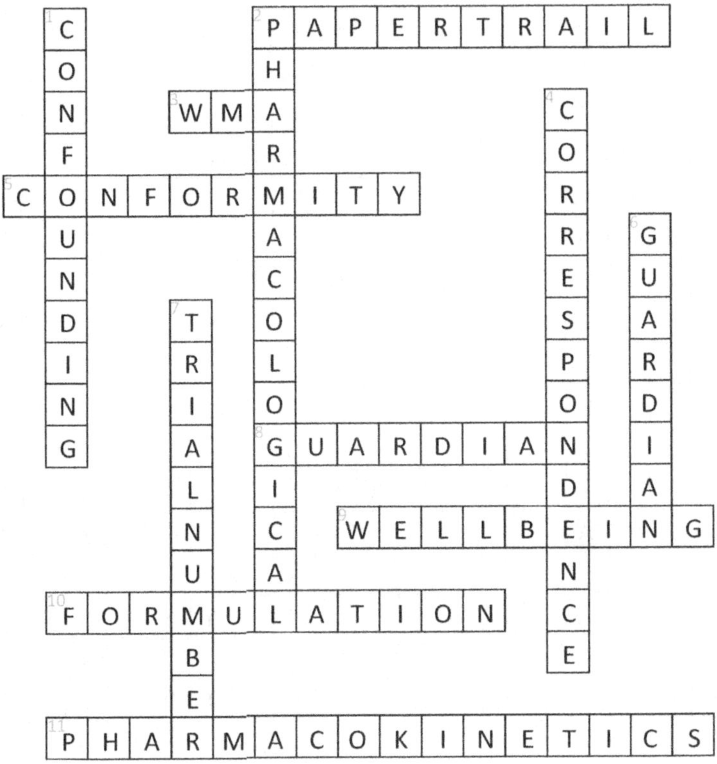

Across

2. PAPER TRAIL
3. WMA
5. CONFORMITY
8. GUARDIAN
9. WELL BEING
10. FORMULATION
11. PHARMACOKINETICS

Down

1. CONFOUNDING
2. PHARMACOLOGICAL
4. CORRESPONDENCE
6. GUARDIAN
7. TRIAL NUMBER

WMA: World Medical Association

Crossword # 109

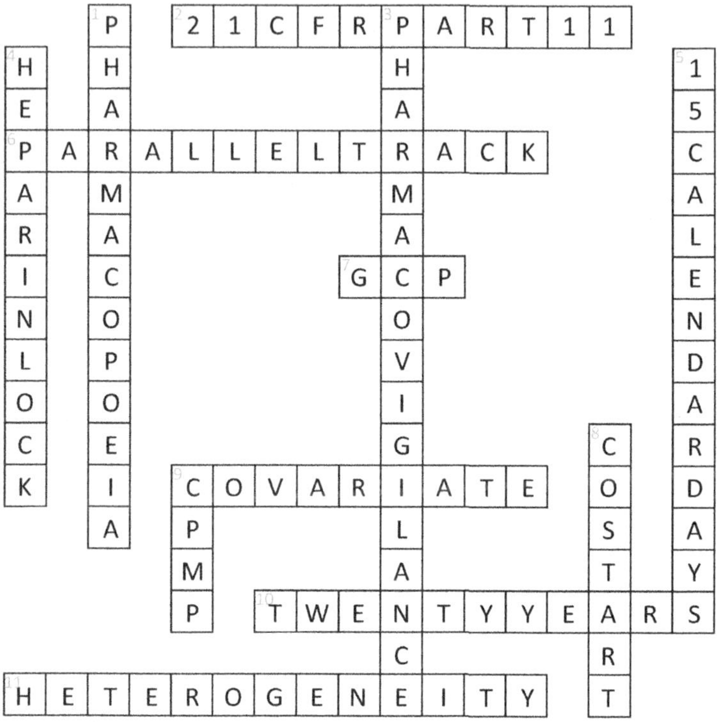

Across

2. 21 CFR PART 11
6. PARALLEL TRACK
7. GCP
9. COVARIATE
10. TWENTY YEARS
11. HETEROGENEITY

Down

1. PHARMACOPOEIA
3. PHARMACOVIGILANCE
4. HEPARIN LOCK
5. 15 CALENDAR DAYS
8. COSTART
9. CPMP

GCP: Good Clinical Practice; **COSTART**: Coding Symbols for a Thesaurus of Adverse Reaction Terms; **CPMP**: Committee for Proprietary Medicinal Products

Crossword # 110

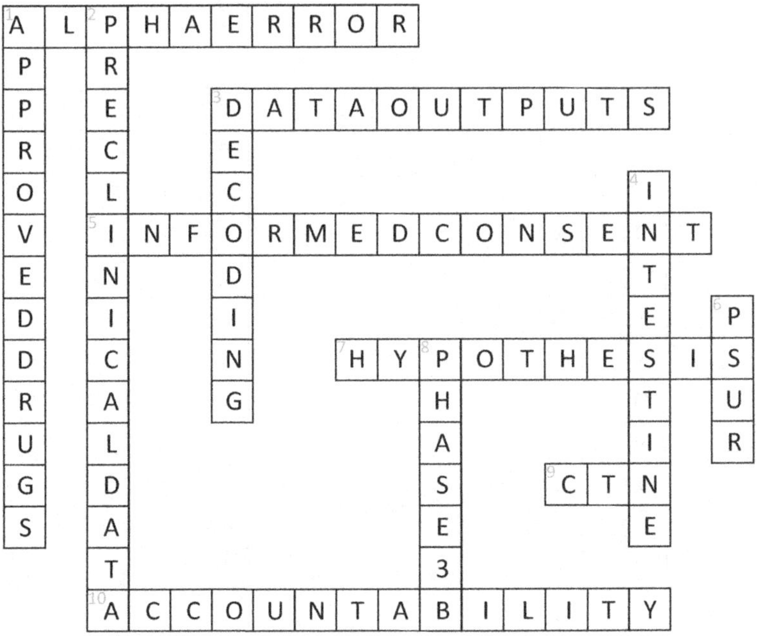

Across

1. ALPHA ERROR
3. DATA OUTPUTS
5. INFORMED CONSENT
7. HYPOTHESIS
9. CTN
10. ACCOUNTABILITY

Down

1. APPROVED DRUGS
2. PRE CLINICAL DATA
3. DECODING
4. INTESTINE
6. PSUR
8. PHASE 3B

PSUR: Periodic Safety Update Report

Crossword # 111

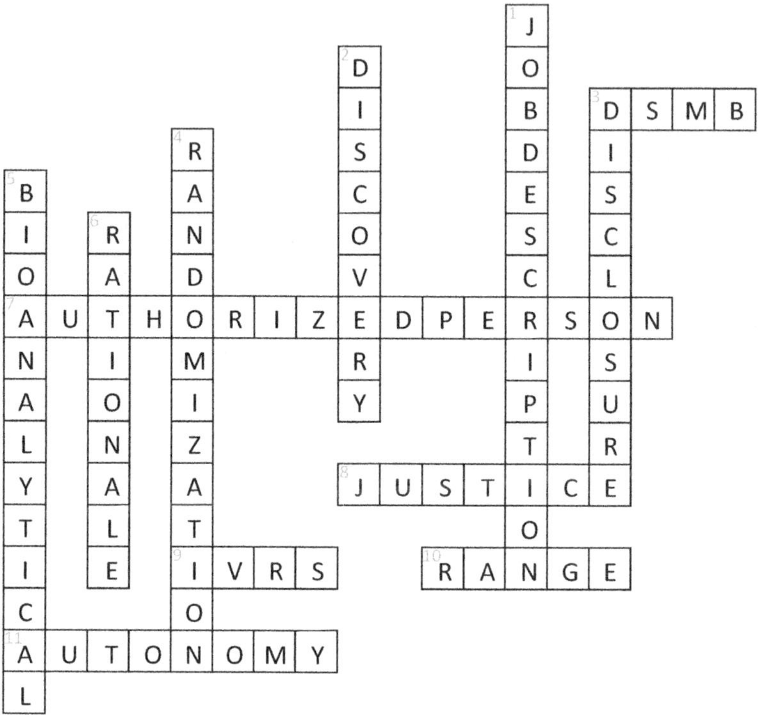

Across

3. DSMB
7. AUTHORIZED PERSON
8. JUSTICE
9. IVRS
10. RANGE
11. AUTONOMY

Down

1. JOB DESCRIPTION
2. DISCOVERY
3. DISCLOSURE
4. RANDOMIZATION
5. BIO ANALYTICAL
6. RATIONALE

DSMB: Data Safety Monitoring Board

Crossword # 112

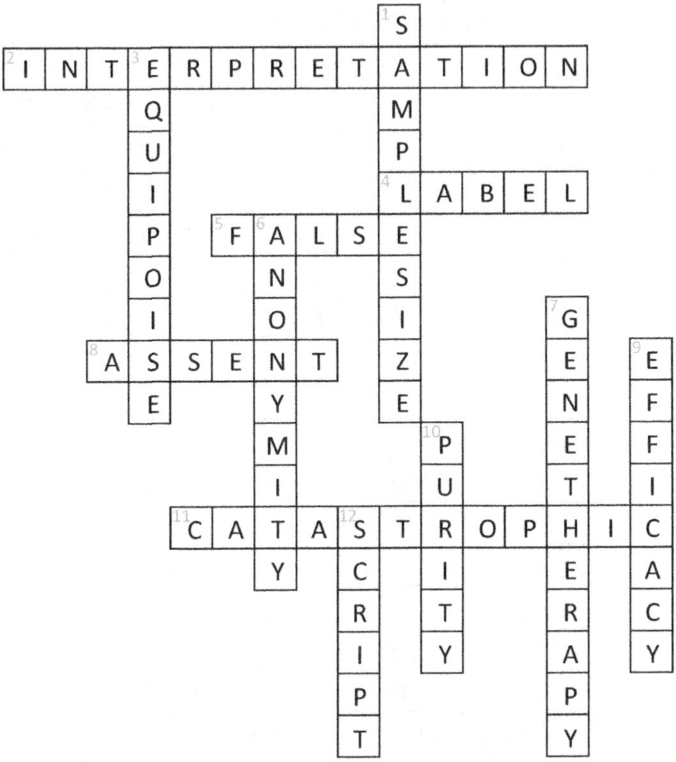

Across

2. INTERPRETATION
4. LABEL
5. FALSE
8. ASSENT
11. CATASTROPHIC

Down

1. SAMPLE SIZE
3. EQUIPOISE
6. ANONYMITY
7. GENE THERAPY
9. EFFICACY
10. PURITY
12. SCRIPT

Crossword # 113

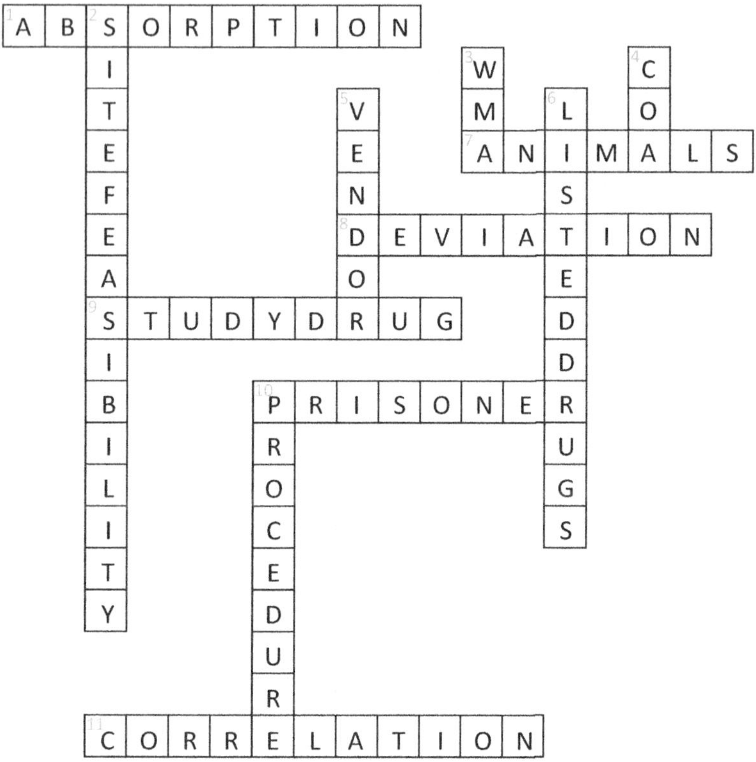

Across

1. ABSORPTION
7. ANIMALS
8. DEVIATION
9. STUDY DRUG
10. PRISONER
11. CORRELATION

Down

2. SITE FEASIBILITY
3. WMA
4. COA
5. VENDOR
6. LISTED DRUGS
10. PROCEDURE

WMA: World Medical Association; **COA**: Certificate of Analysis

Crossword # 114

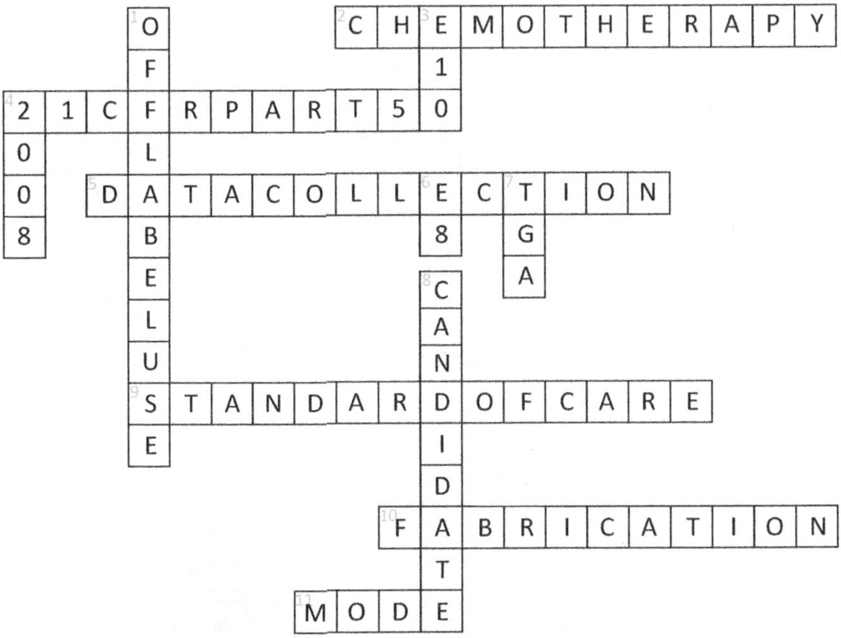

Across

2. CHEMOTHERAPY
4. 21 CFR PART 50
5. DATA COLLECTION
9. STANDARD OF CARE
10. FABRICATION
11. MODE

Down

1. OFF LABEL USE
3. E10
4. 2008
6. E8
7. TGA
8. CANDIDATE

TGA: Therapeutics Goods Administration

Crossword # 115

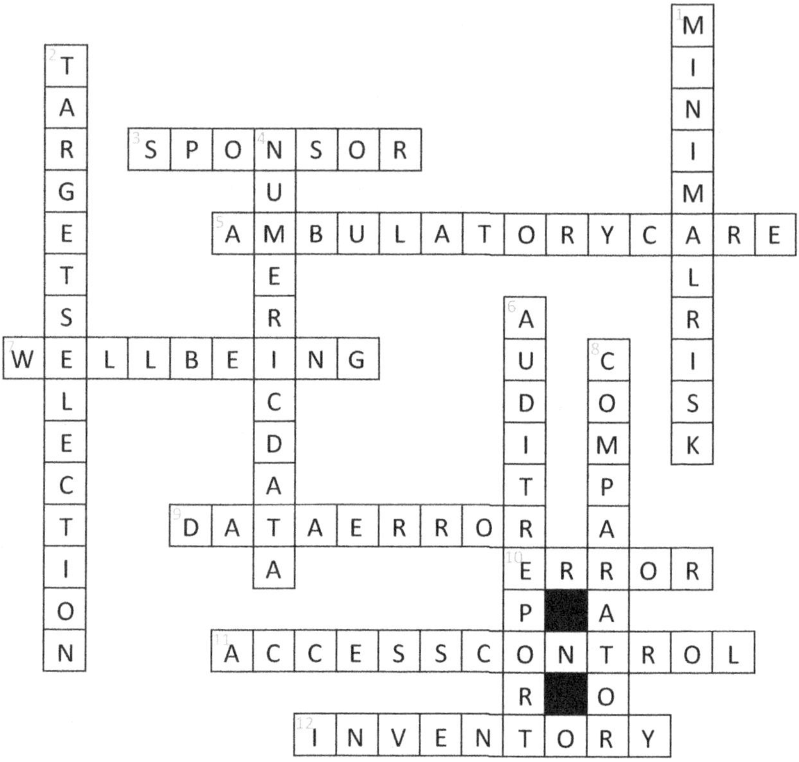

Across

3. SPONSOR
5. AMBULATORY CARE
7. WELL BEING
9. DATA ERROR
10. ERROR
11. ACCESS CONTROL
12. INVENTORY

Down

1. MINIMAL RISK
2. TARGET SELECTION
4. NUMERIC DATA
6. AUDIT REPORT
8. COMPARATOR

Crossword # 116

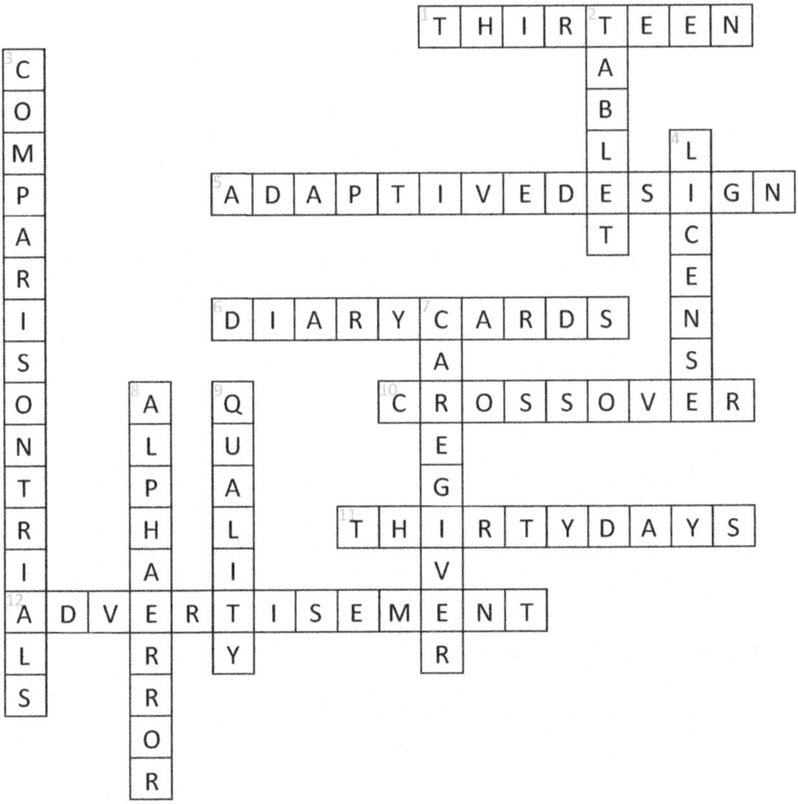

Across

1. THIRTEEN
5. ADAPTIVE DESIGN
6. DIARY CARDS
10. CROSS OVER
11. THIRTY DAYS
12. ADVERTISEMENT

Down

2. TABLET
3. COMPARISON TRIALS
4. LICENSE
7. CARE GIVER
8. ALPHA ERROR
9. QUALITY

Crossword # 117

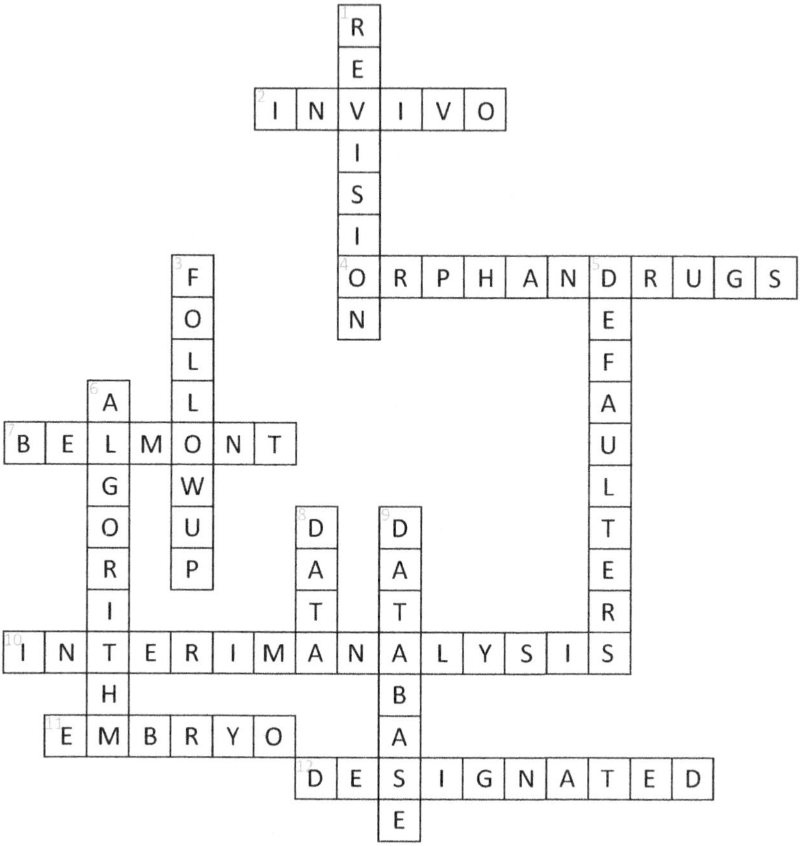

Across

2. IN VIVO
4. ORPHAN DRUGS
7. BELMONT
10. INTERIM ANALYSIS
11. EMBRYO
12. DESIGNATED

Down

1. REVISION
3. FOLLOW UP
5. DEFAULTERS
6. ALGORITHM
8. DATA
9. DATABASE

Crossword # 118

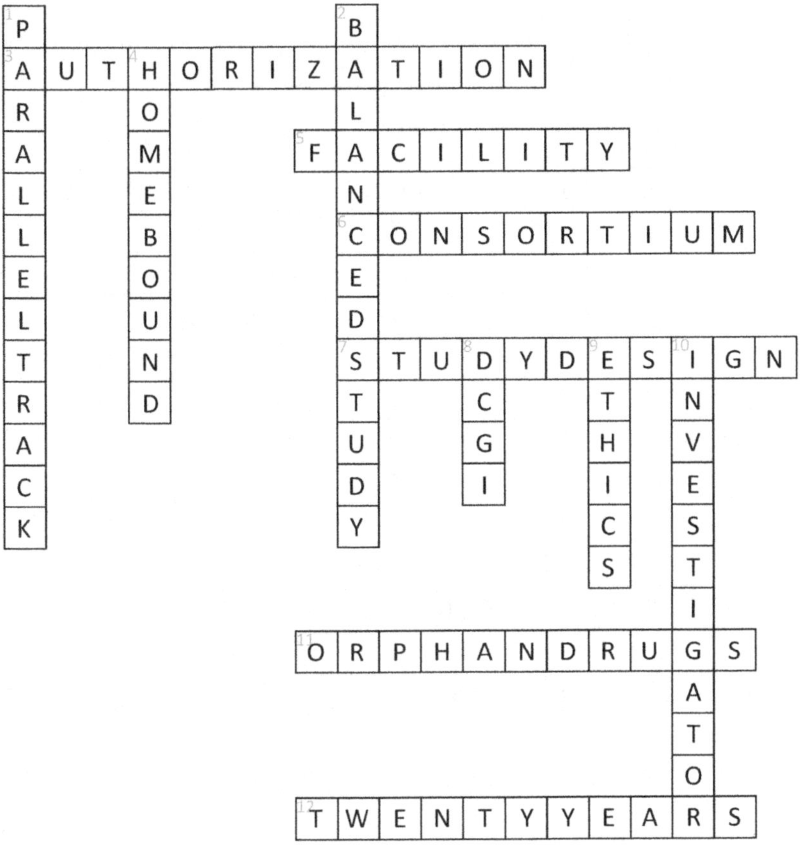

Across

3. AUTHORIZATION
5. FACILITY
6. CONSORTIUM
7. STUDY DESIGN
11. ORPHAN DRUGS
12. TWENTY YEARS

Down

1. PARALLEL TRACK
2. BALANCED STUDY
4. HOME BOUND
8. DCGI
9. ETHICS
10. INVESTIGATOR

DCGI: Drug Controller General of India

Crossword # 119

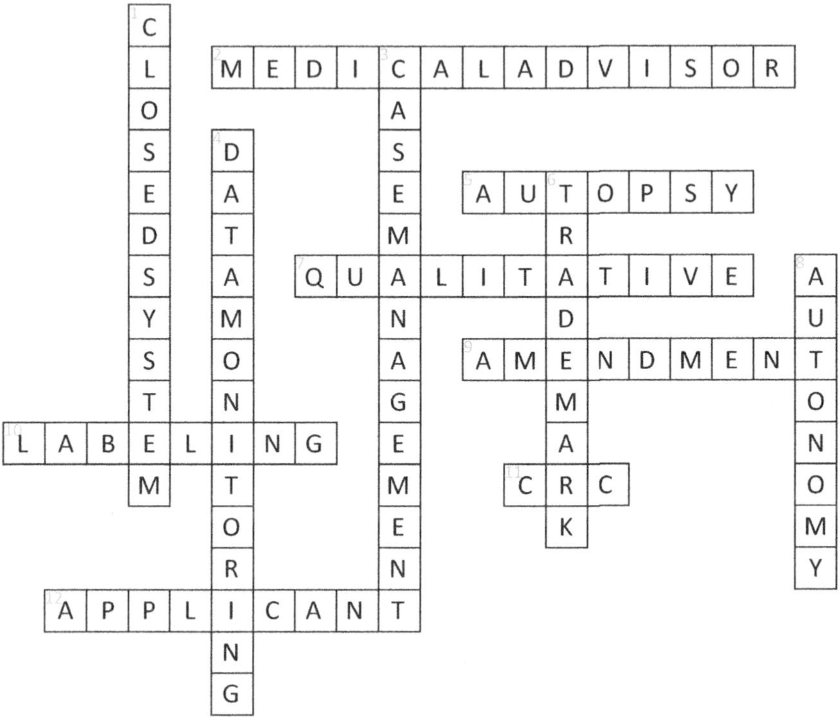

Across

2. MEDICAL ADVISOR
5. AUTOPSY
7. QUALITATIVE
9. AMENDMENT
10. LABELING
11. CRC
12. APPLICANT

Down

1. CLOSED SYSTEM
3. CASE MANAGEMENT
4. DATA MONITORING
6. TRADEMARK
8. AUTONOMY

CRC: Clinical Research Coordinator

Crossword # 120

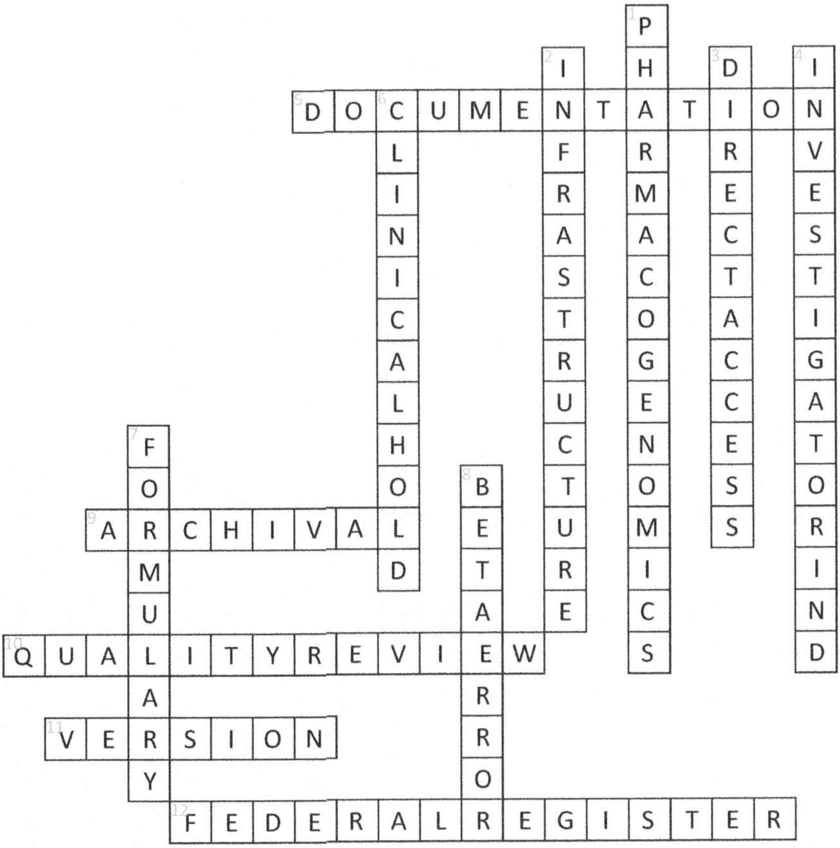

Across

5. DOCUMENTATION
9. ARCHIVAL
10. QUALITY REVIEW
11. VERSION
12. FEDERAL REGISTER

Down

1. PHARMACOGENOMICS
2. INFRASTRUCTURE
3. DIRECT ACCESS
4. INVESTIGATOR IND
6. CLINICAL HOLD
7. FORMULARY
8. BETA ERROR

Crossword # 121

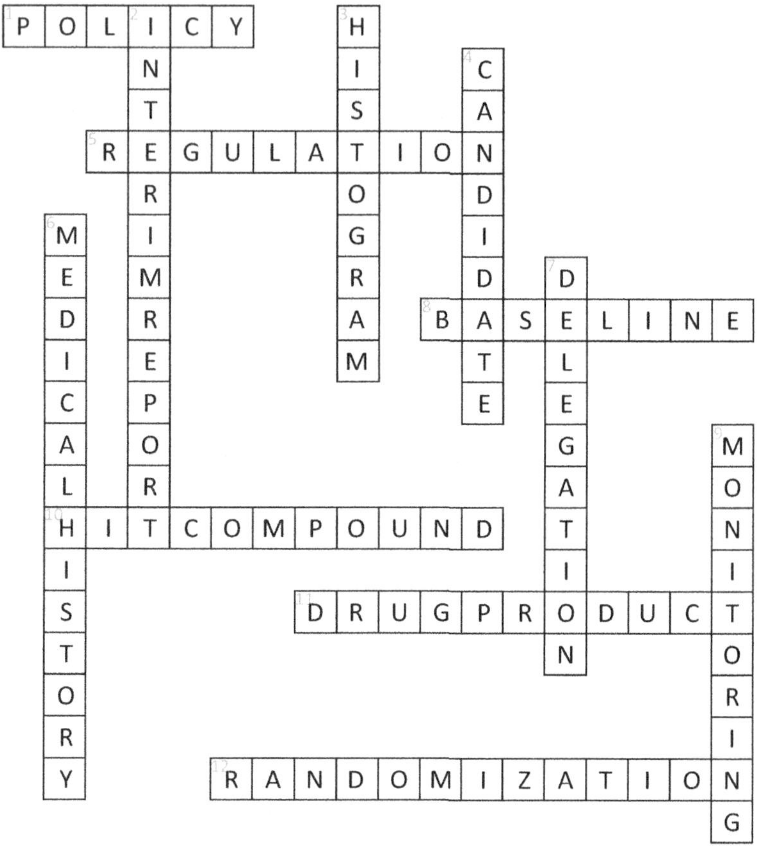

Across

1. POLICY
5. REGULATION
8. BASELINE
10. HIT COMPOUND
11. DRUG PRODUCT
12. RANDOMIZATION

Down

2. INTERIM REPORT
3. HISTOGRAM
4. CANDIDATE
6. MEDICAL HISTORY
7. DELEGATION
9. MONITORING

Crossword # 122

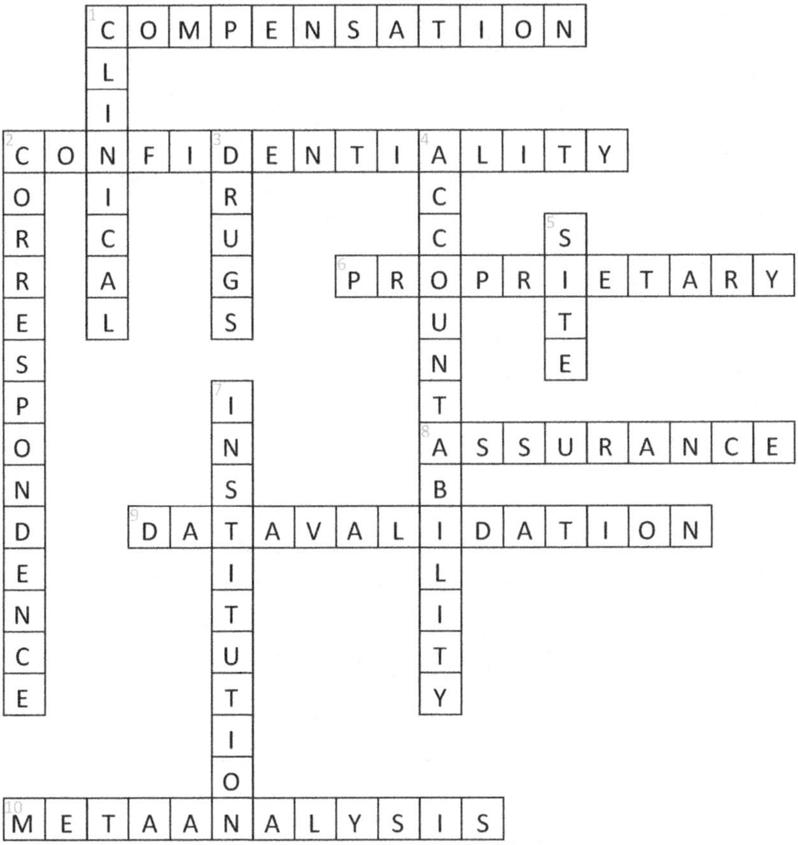

Across

1. COMPENSATION
2. CONFIDENTIALITY
6. PROPRIETARY
8. ASSURANCE
9. DATA VALIDATION
10. META ANALYSIS

Down

1. CLINICAL
2. CORRESPONDENCE
3. DRUGS
4. ACCOUNTABILITY
5. SITE
7. INSTITUTION

Crossword # 123

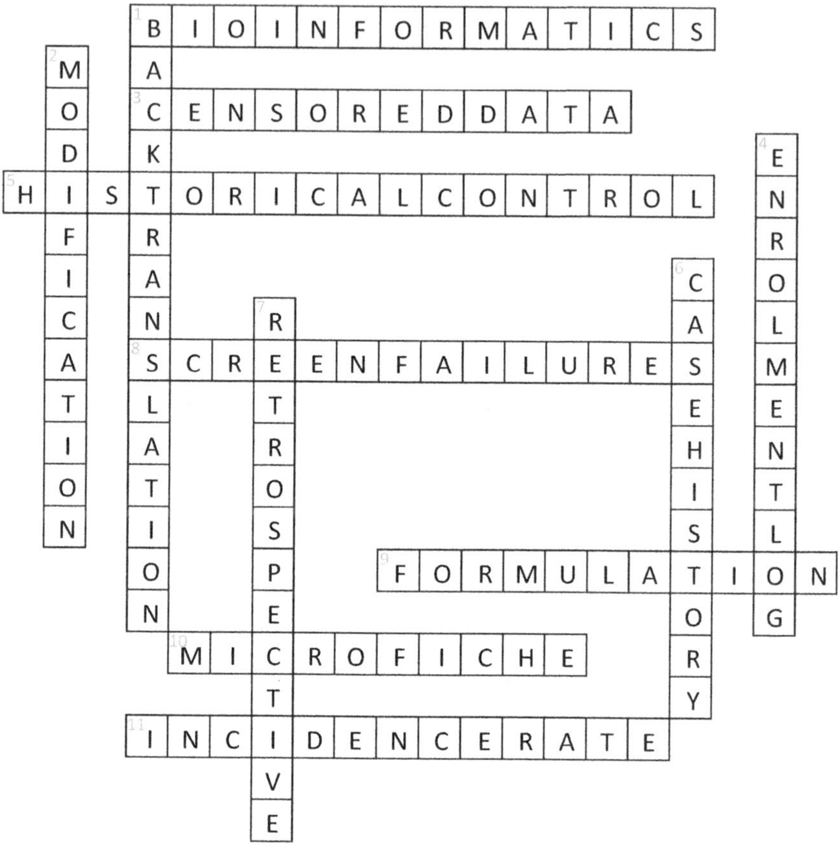

Across

1. BIOINFORMATICS
3. CENSORED DATA
5. HISTORICAL CONTROL
8. SCREEN FAILURES
9. FORMULATION
10. MICROFICHE
11. INCIDENCE RATE

Down

1. BACK TRANSLATION
2. MODIFICATION
4. ENROLMENT LOG
6. CASE HISTORY
7. RETROSPECTIVE

Crossword # 124

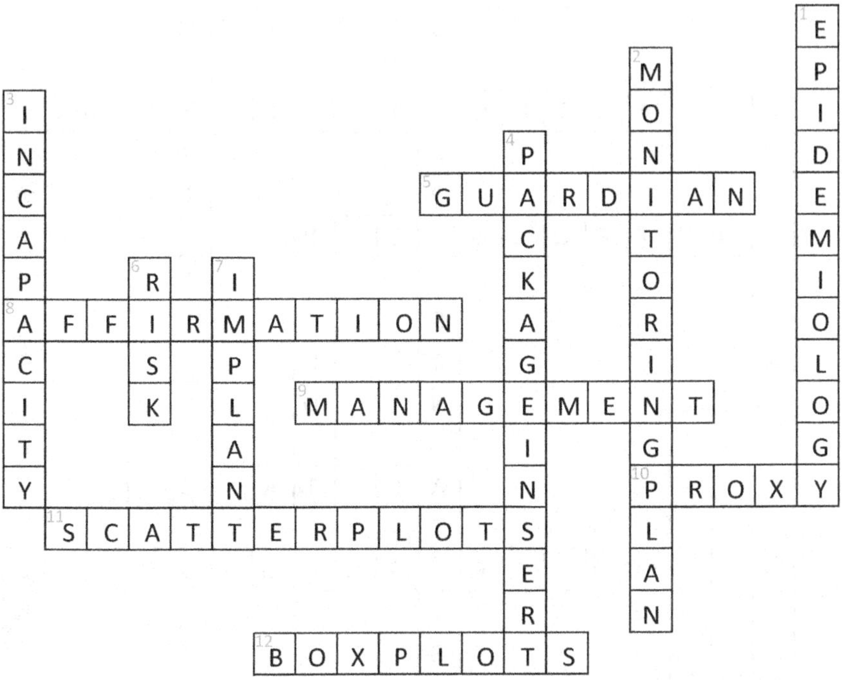

Across

5. GUARDIAN
8. AFFIRMATION
9. MANAGEMENT
10. PROXY
11. SCATTER PLOTS
12. BOX PLOTS

Down

1. EPIDEMIOLOGY
2. MONITORING PLAN
3. INCAPACITY
4. PACKAGE INSERT
6. RISK
7. IMPLANT

Crossword # 125

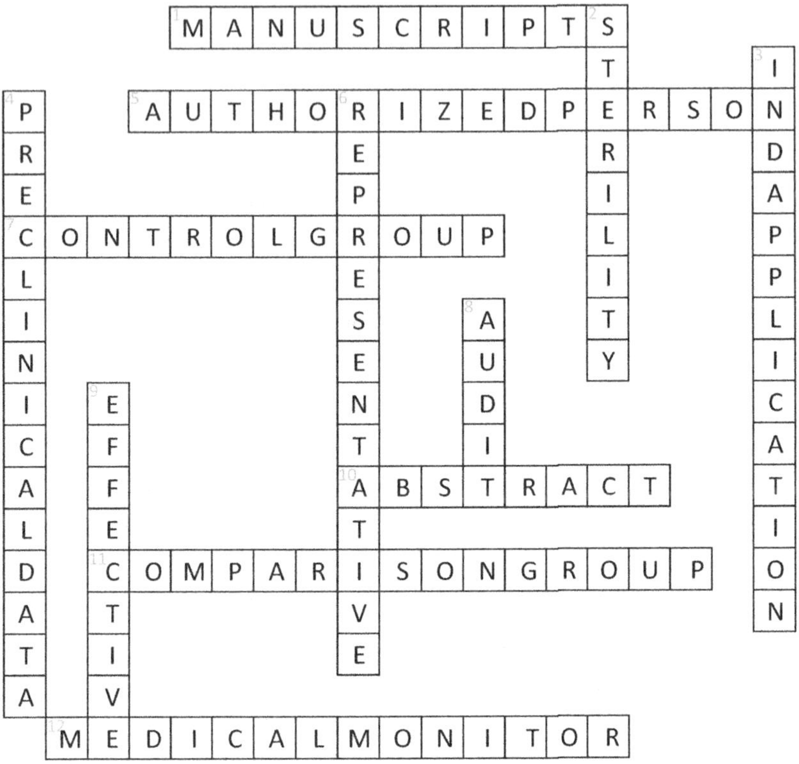

Across

1. MANUSCRIPTS
5. AUTHORIZED PERSON
7. CONTROL GROUP
10. ABSTRACT
11. COMPARISON GROUP
12. MEDICAL MONITOR

Down

2. STERILITY
3. IND APPLICATION
4. PRE CLINICAL DATA
6. REPRESENTATIVE
8. AUDIT
9. EFFECTIVE

Crossword # 126

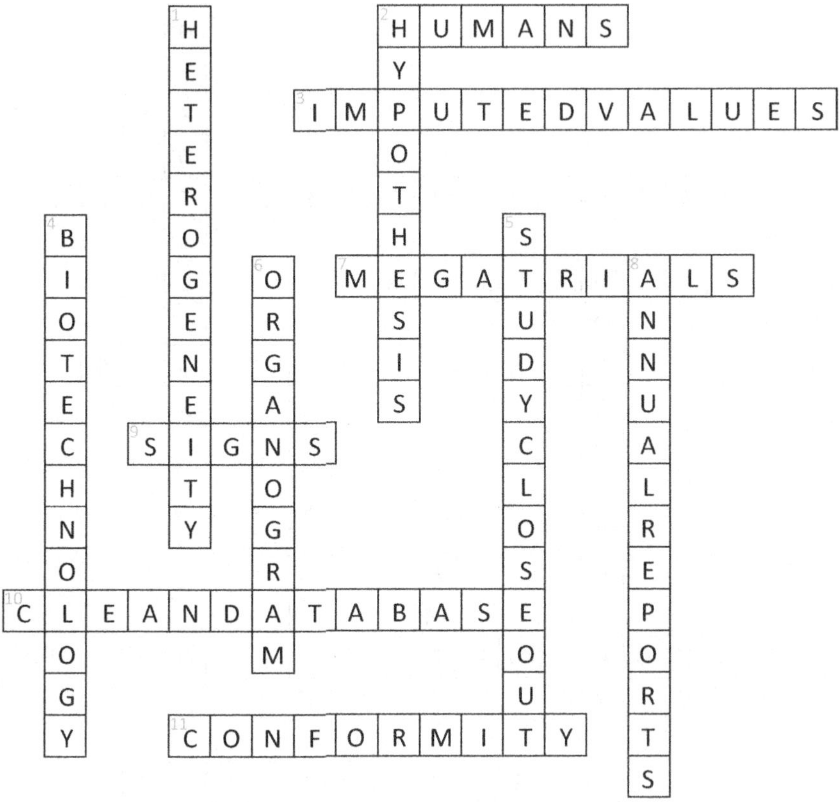

Across

2. HUMANS
3. IMPUTED VALUES
7. MEGA TRIALS
9. SIGNS
10. CLEAN DATABASE
11. CONFORMITY

Down

1. HETEROGENEITY
2. HYPOTHESIS
4. BIOTECHNOLOGY
5. STUDY CLOSEOUT
6. ORGANOGRAM
8. ANNUAL REPORTS

Crossword # 127

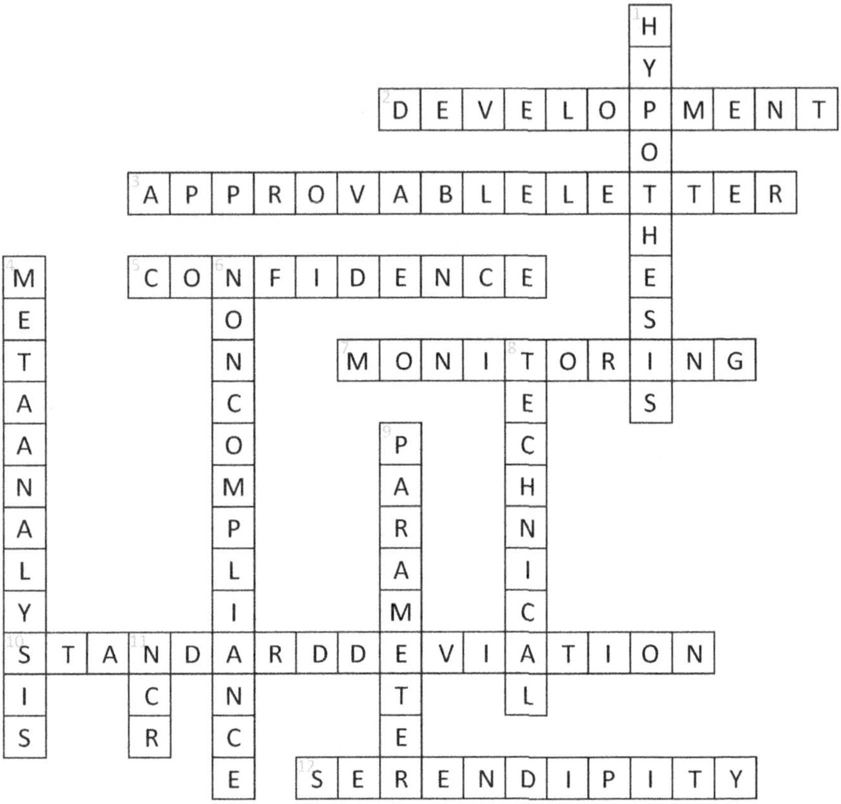

Across

2. DEVELOPMENT
3. APPROVABLE LETTER
5. CONFIDENCE
7. MONITORING
10. STANDARD DEVIATION
12. SERENDIPITY

Down

1. HYPOTHESIS
4. META ANALYSIS
6. NON COMPLIANCE
8. TECHNICAL
9. PARAMETER
11. NCR

NCR: No Carbon Required

Crossword # 128

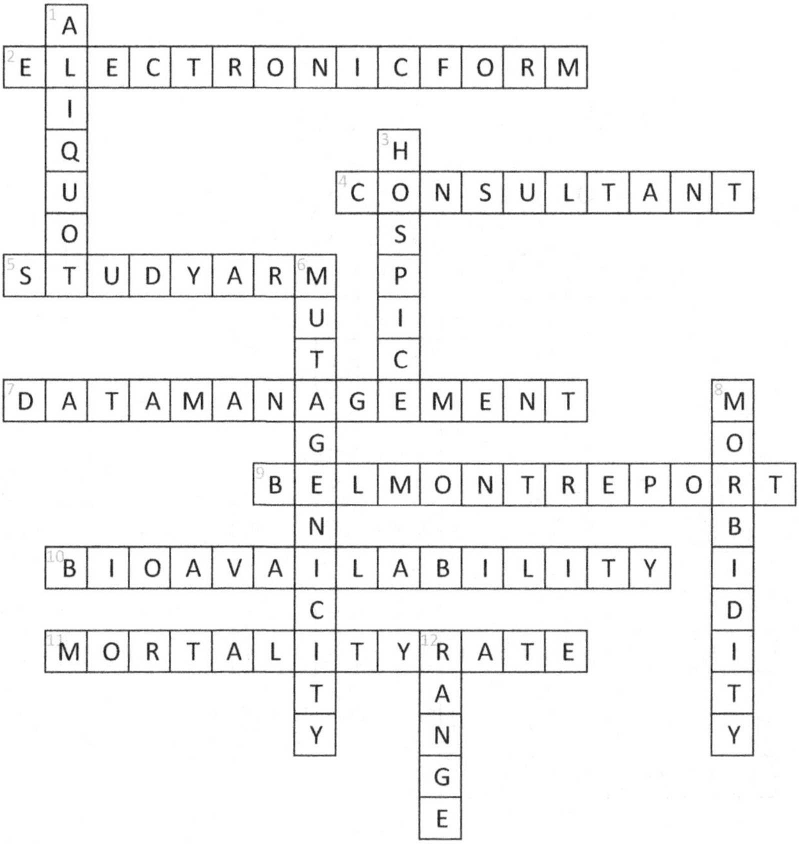

Across

2. ELECTRONIC FORM
4. CONSULTANT
5. STUDY ARM
7. DATA MANAGEMENT
9. BELMONT REPORT
10. BIOAVAILABILITY
11. MORTALITY RATE

Down

1. ALIQUOT
3. HOSPICE
6. MUTAGENICITY
8. MORBIDITY
12. RANGE

Crossword # 129

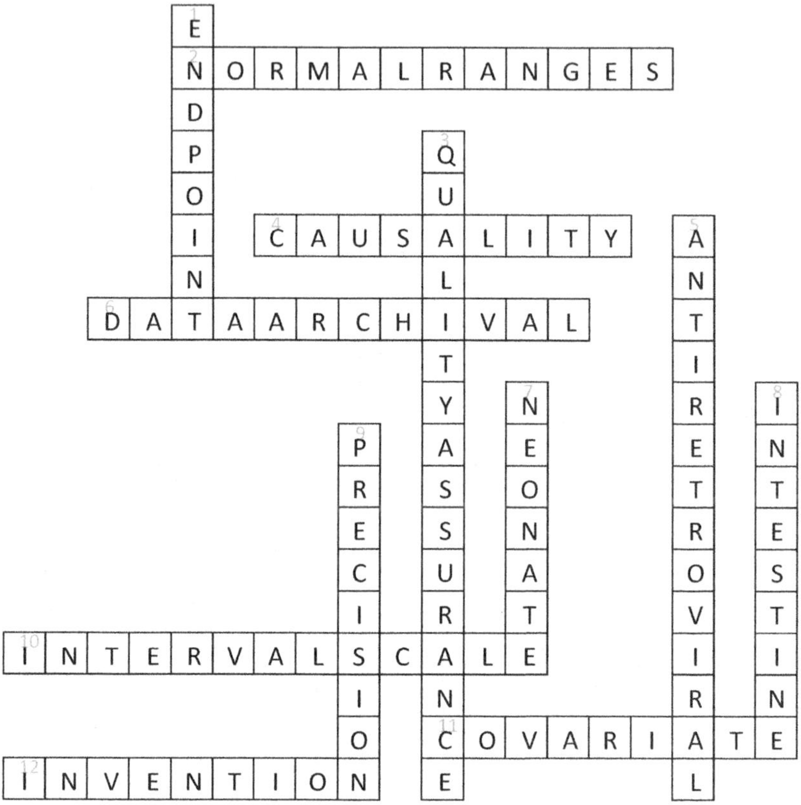

Across

2. NORMAL RANGES
4. CAUSALITY
6. DATA ARCHIVAL
10. INTERVAL SCALE
11. COVARIATE
12. INVENTION

Down

1. ENDPOINT
3. QUALITY ASSURANCE
5. ANTIRETROVIRAL
7. NEONATE
8. INTESTINE
9. PRECISION

Crossword # 130

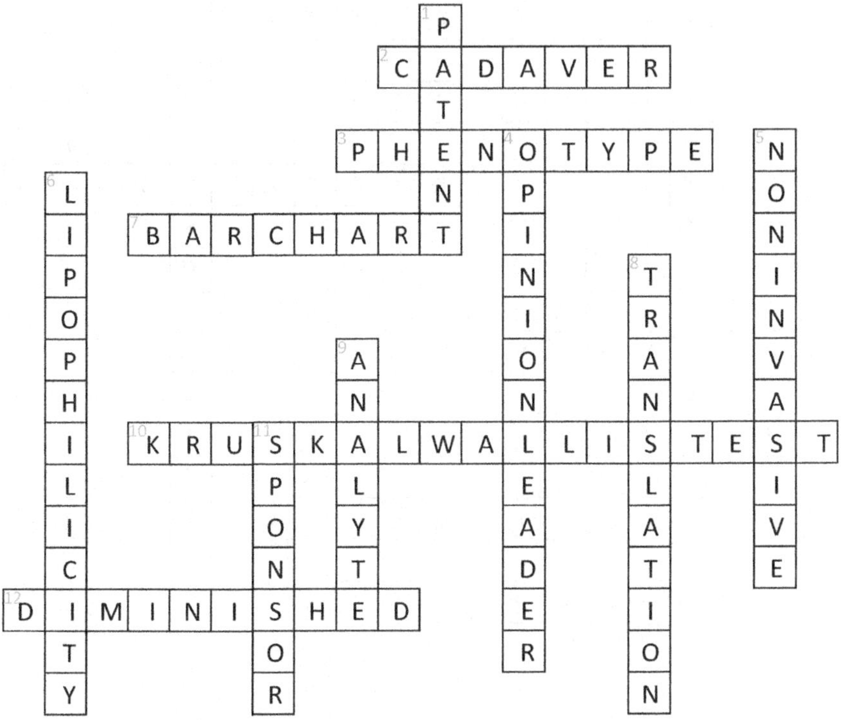

Across

2. CADAVER
3. PHENOTYPE
7. BAR CHART
10. KRUSKAL WALLIS TEST
12. DIMINISHED

Down

1. PATENT
4. OPINION LEADER
5. NON INVASIVE
6. LIPOPHILICITY
8. TRANSLATION
9. ANALYTE
11. SPONSOR

Crossword # 131

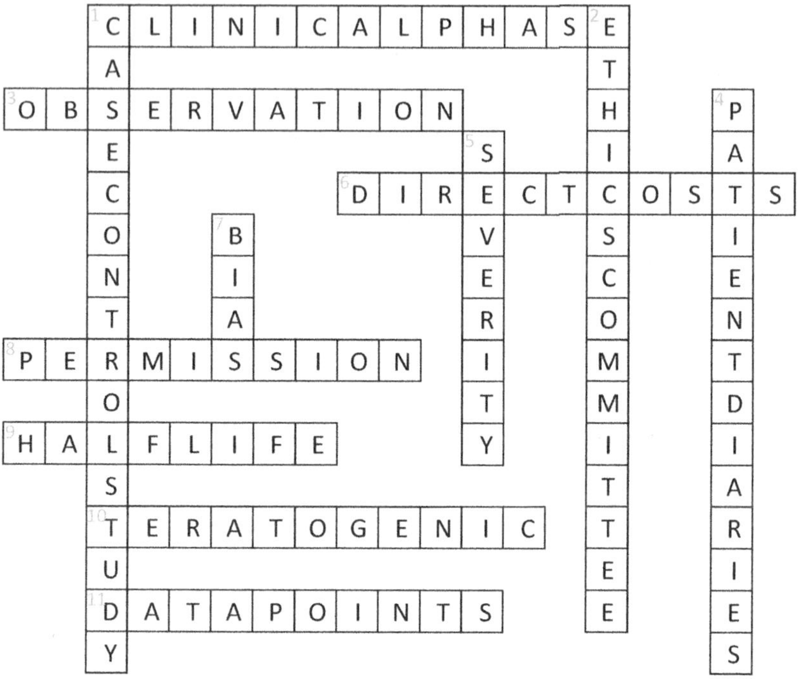

Across

1. CLINICAL PHASE
3. OBSERVATION
6. DIRECT COSTS
8. PERMISSION
9. HALF LIFE
10. TERATOGENIC
11. DATA POINTS

Down

1. CASE CONTROL STUDY
2. ETHICS COMMITTEE
4. PATIENT DIARIES
5. SEVERITY
7. BIAS

Crossword # 132

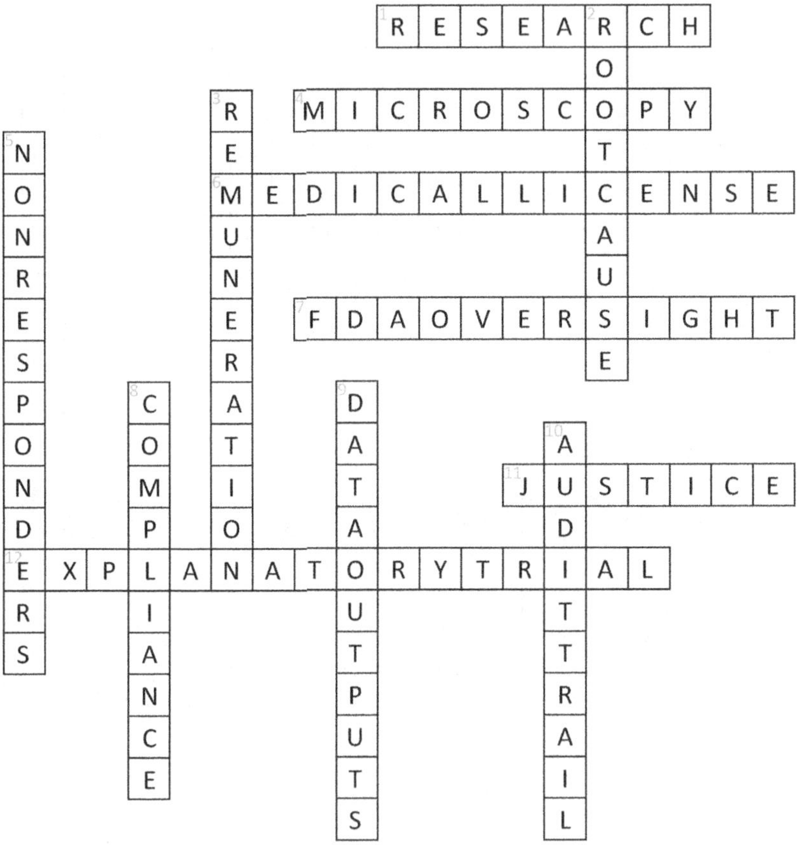

Across

1. RESEARCH
4. MICROSCOPY
6. MEDICAL LICENSE
7. FDA OVERSIGHT
11. JUSTICE
12. EXPLANATORY TRIAL

Down

2. ROOT CAUSE
3. REMUNERATION
5. NON RESPONDERS
8. COMPLIANCE
9. DATA OUTPUTS
10. AUDIT TRAIL

Crossword # 133

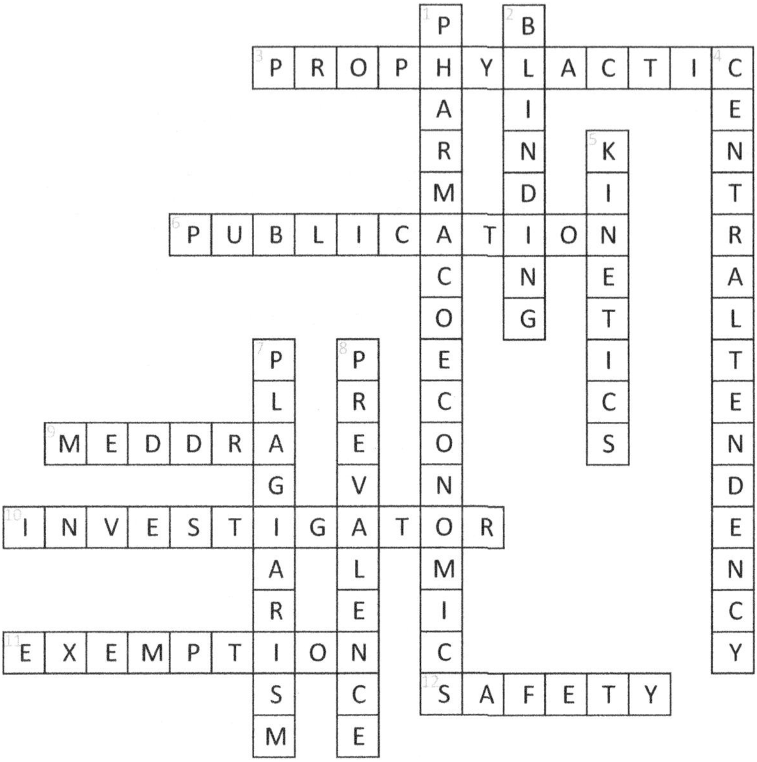

Across

3. PROPHYLACTIC
6. PUBLICATION
9. MedDRA
10. INVESTIGATOR
11. EXEMPTION
12. SAFETY

Down

1. PHARMACOECONOMICS
2. BLINDING
4. CENTRAL TENDENCY
5. KINETICS
7. PLAGIARISM
8. PREVALENCE

MedDRA: Medical Dictionary for Regulatory Activities

Crossword # 134

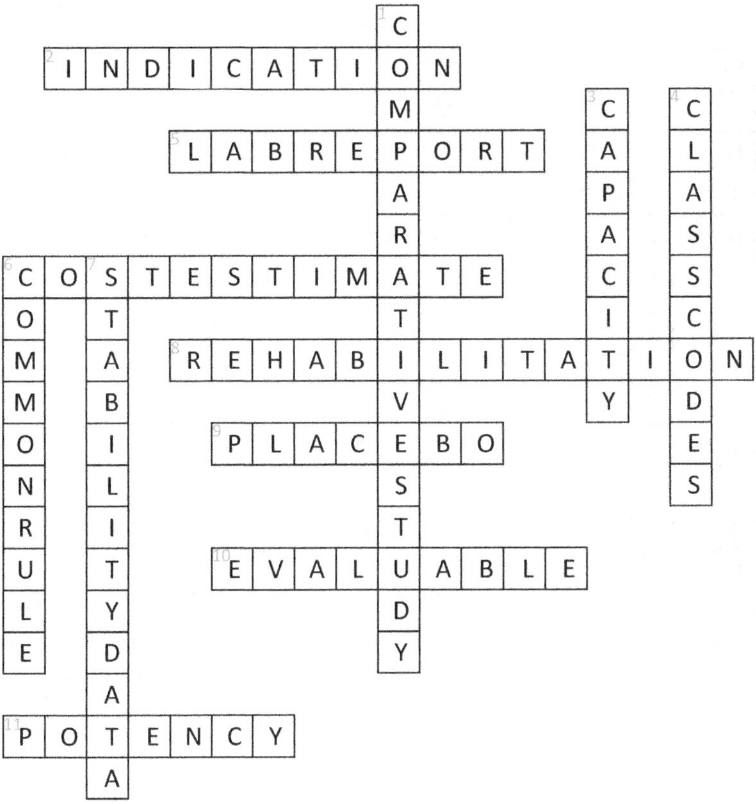

Across

2. INDICATION
5. LAB REPORT
6. COST ESTIMATE
8. REHABILITATION
9. PLACEBO
10. EVALUABLE
11. POTENCY

Down

1. COMPARATIVE STUDY
3. CAPACITY
4. CLASS CODES
6. COMMON RULE
7. STABILITY DATA

Crossword # 135

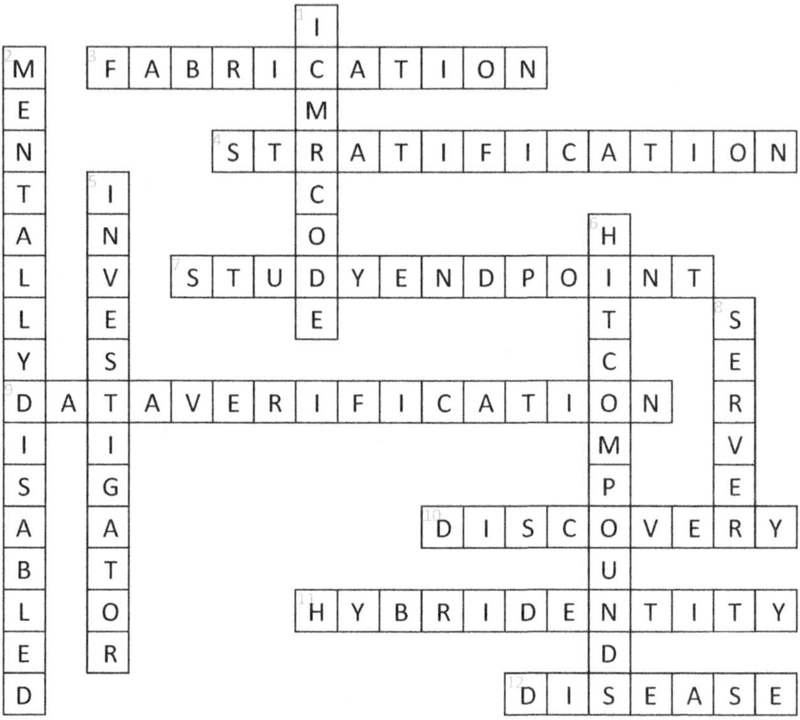

Across

3. FABRICATION
4. STRATIFICATION
7. STUDY ENDPOINT
9. DATA VERIFICATION
10. DISCOVERY
11. HYBRID ENTITY
12. DISEASE

Down

1. ICMR CODE
2. MENTALLY DISABLED
5. INVESTIGATOR
6. HIT COMPOUNDS
8. SERVER

Crossword # 136

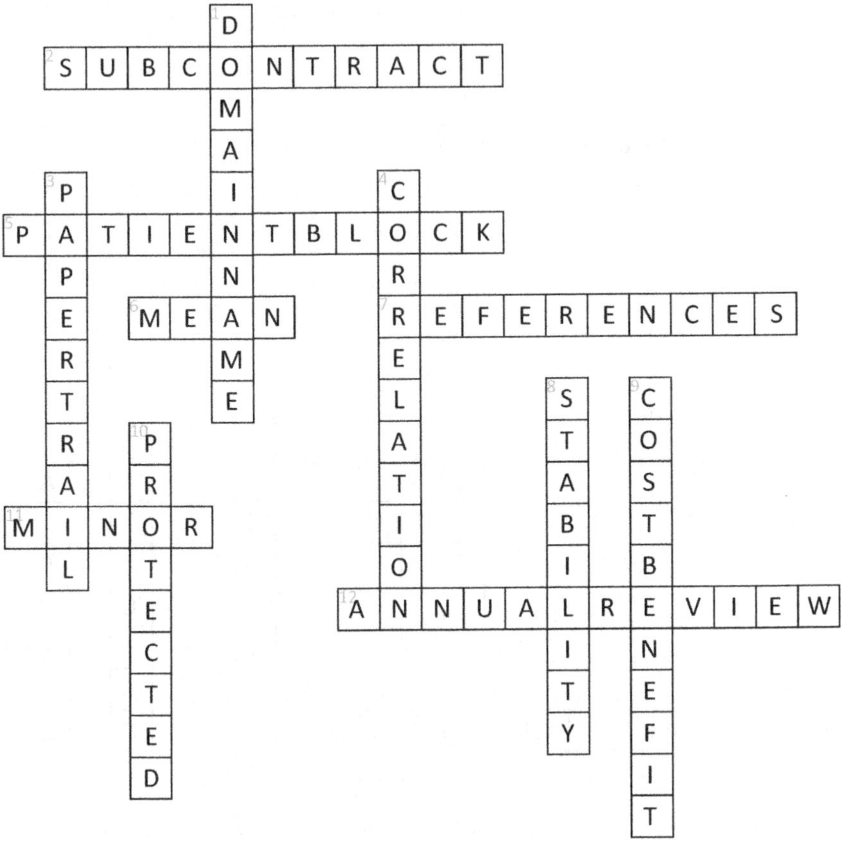

Across

2. SUB CONTRACT
5. PATIENT BLOCK
6. MEAN
7. REFERENCES
11. MINOR
12. ANNUAL REVIEW

Down

1. DOMAIN NAME
3. PAPER TRAIL
4. CORRELATION
8. STABILITY
9. COST BENEFIT
10. PROTECTED

Crossword # 137

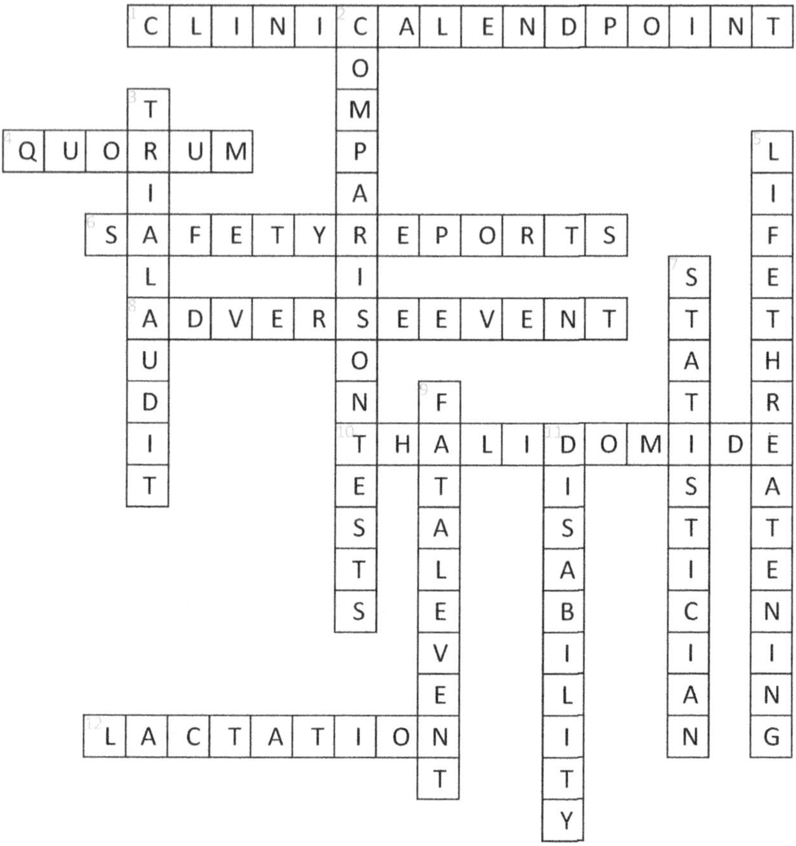

Across

1. CLINICAL ENDPOINT
4. QUORUM
6. SAFETY REPORTS
8. ADVERSE EVENT
10. THALIDOMIDE
12. LACTATION

Down

2. COMPARISON TESTS
3. TRIAL AUDIT
5. LIFE THREATENING
7. STATISTICIAN
9. FATAL EVENT
11. DISABILITY

Crossword # 138

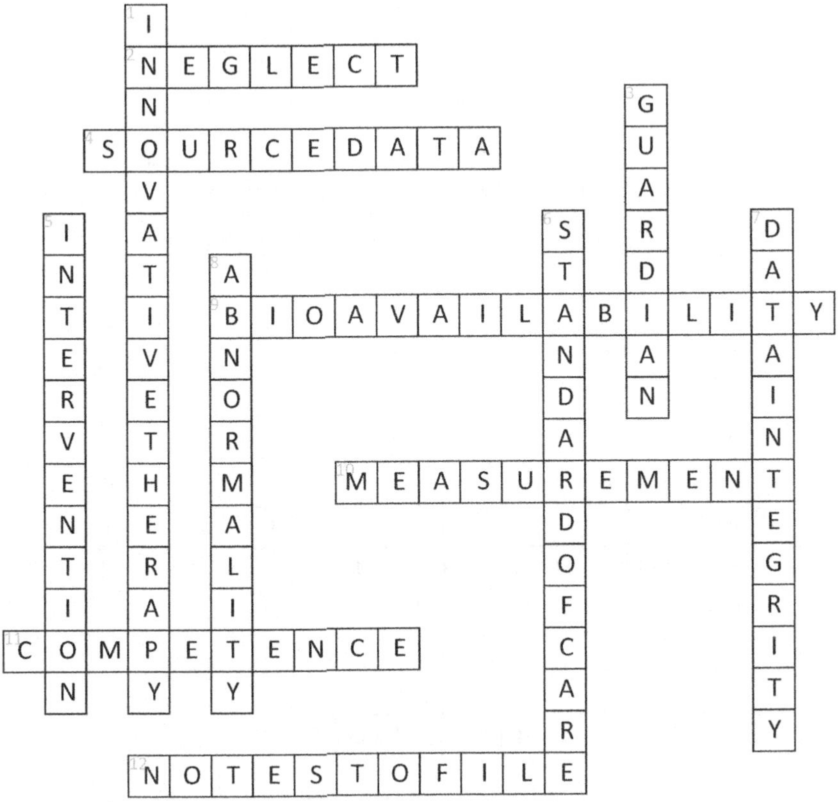

Across

2. NEGLECT
4. SOURCE DATA
9. BIOAVAILABILITY
10. MEASUREMENT
11. COMPETENCE
12. NOTES TO FILE

Down

1. INNOVATIVE THERAPY
3. GUARDIAN
5. INTERVENTION
6. STANDARD OF CARE
7. DATA INTEGRITY
8. ABNORMALITY

Crossword # 139

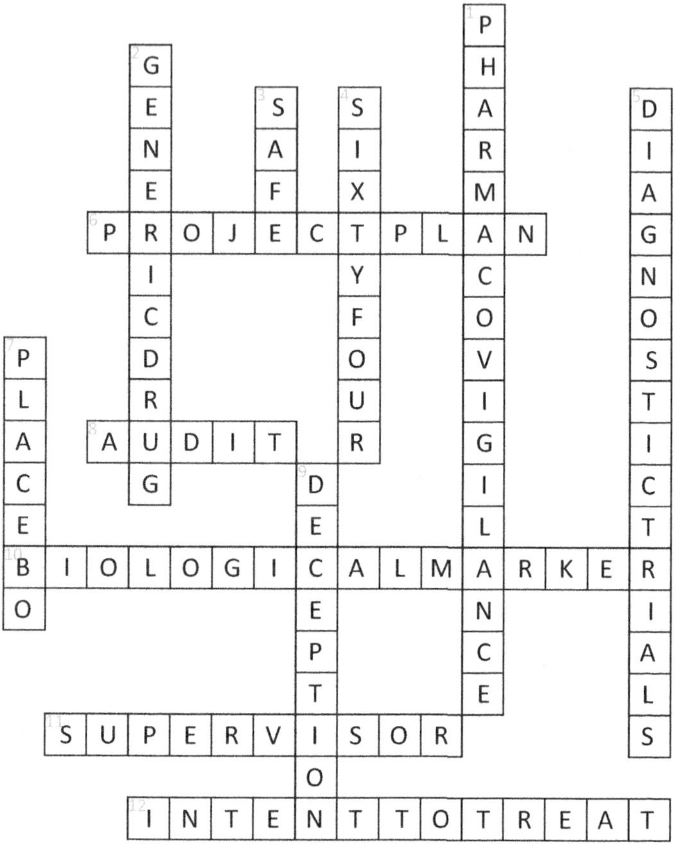

Across

6. PROJECT PLAN
8. AUDIT
10. BIOLOGICAL MARKER
11. SUPERVISOR
12. INTENT TO TREAT

Down

1. PHARMACOVIGILANCE
2. GENERIC DRUG
3. SAFE
4. SIXTY FOUR
5. DIAGNOSTIC TRIALS
7. PLACEBO
9. DECEPTION

Crossword # 140

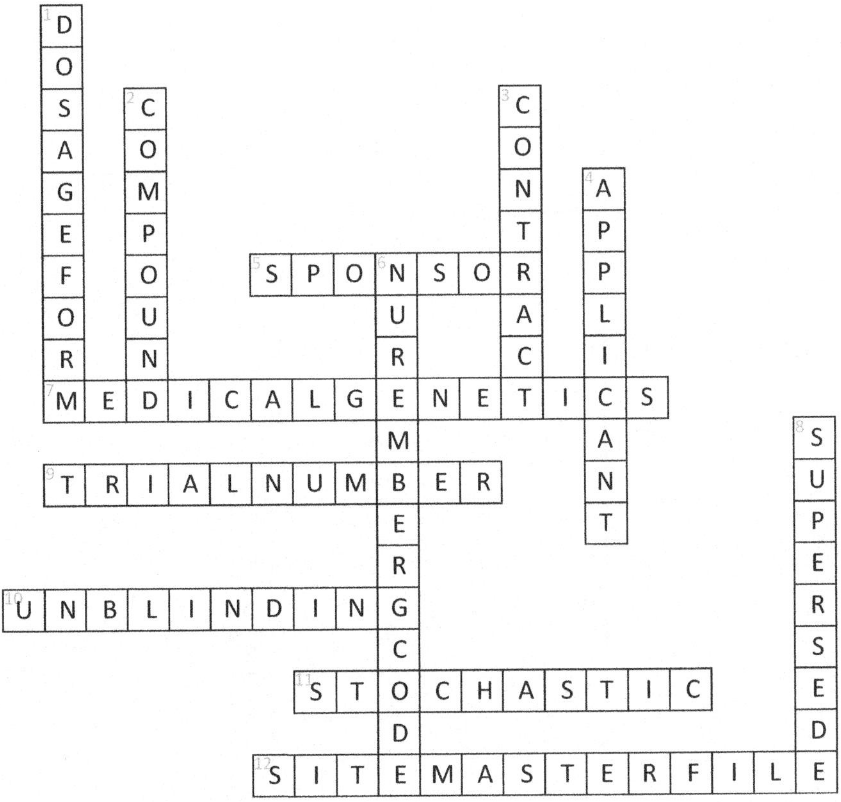

Across

5. SPONSOR
7. MEDICAL GENETICS
9. TRIAL NUMBER
10. UNBLINDING
11. STOCHASTIC
12. SITE MASTER FILE

Down

1. DOSAGE FORM
2. COMPOUND
3. CONTRACT
4. APPLICANT
6. NUREMBERG CODE
8. SUPERSEDE

Crossword # 141

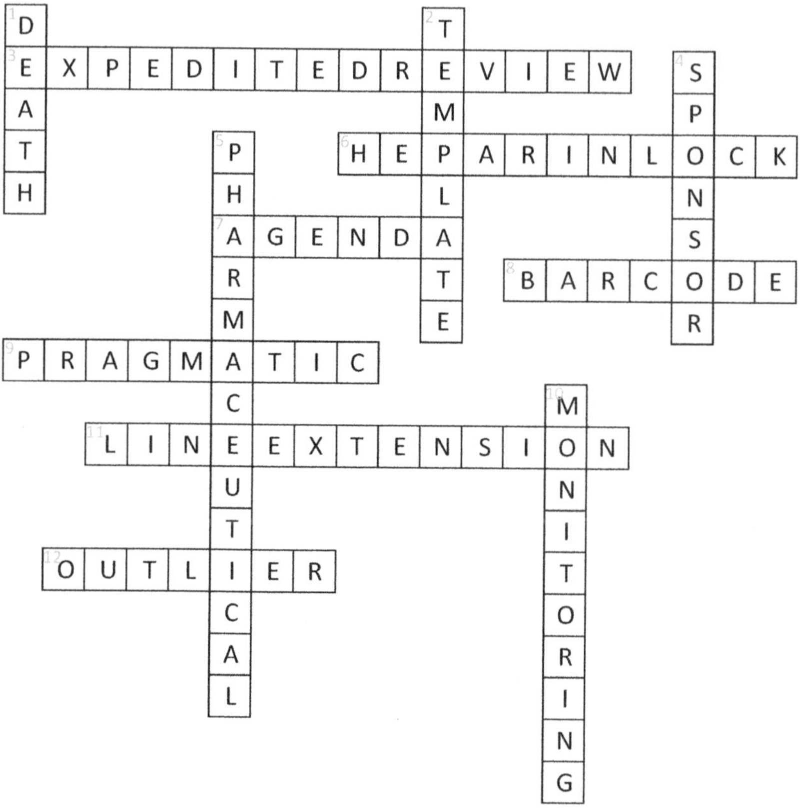

Across

3. EXPEDITED REVIEW
6. HEPARIN LOCK
7. AGENDA
8. BARCODE
9. PRAGMATIC
11. LINE EXTENSION
12. OUTLIER

Down

1. DEATH
2. TEMPLATE
4. SPONSOR
5. PHARMACEUTICAL
10. MONITORING

Crossword # 142

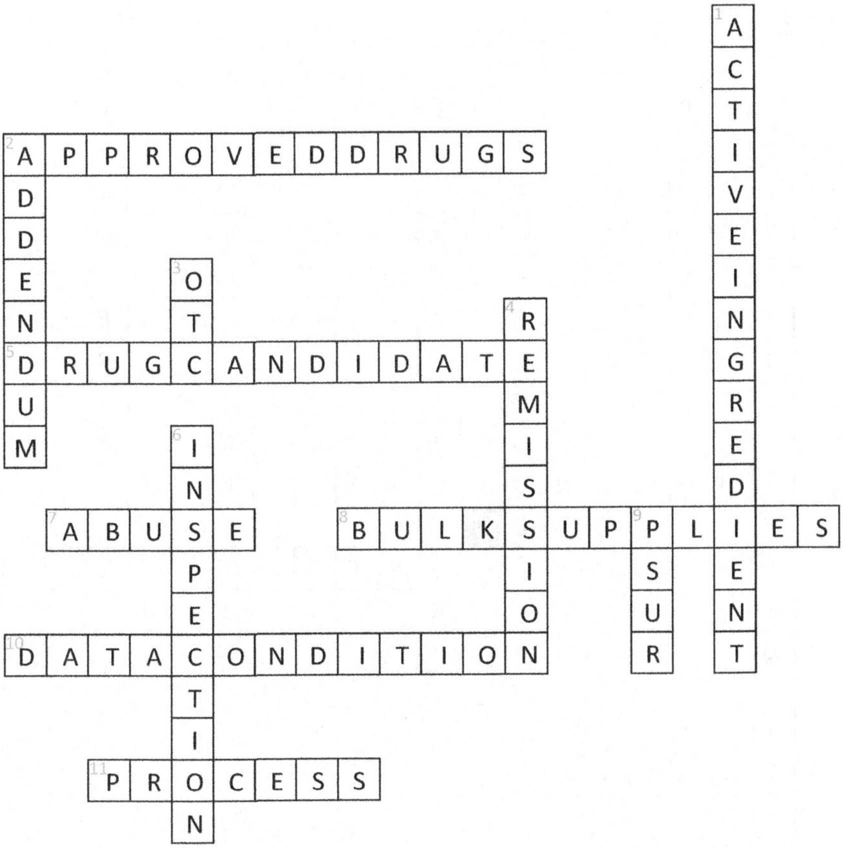

Across

2. APPROVED DRUGS
5. DRUG CANDIDATE
7. ABUSE
8. BULK SUPPLIES
10. DATA CONDITION
11. PROCESS

Down

1. ACTIVE INGREDIENT
2. ADDENDUM
3. OTC
4. REMISSION
6. INSPECTION
9. PSUR

OTC: Over The Counter; **PSUR**: Periodic Safety Update Report

Crossword # 143

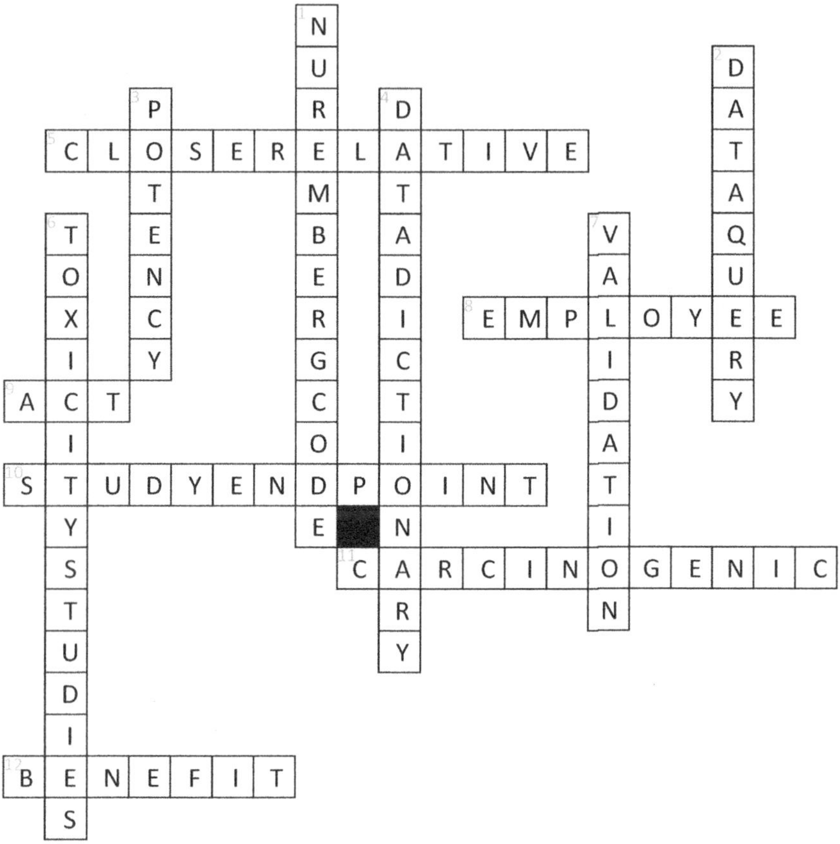

Across

5. CLOSE RELATIVE
8. EMPLOYEE
9. ACT
10. STUDY ENDPOINT
11. CARCINOGENIC
12. BENEFIT

Down

1. NUREMBERG CODE
2. DATA QUERY
3. POTENCY
4. DATA DICTIONARY
6. TOXICITY STUDIES
7. VALIDATION

Crossword # 144

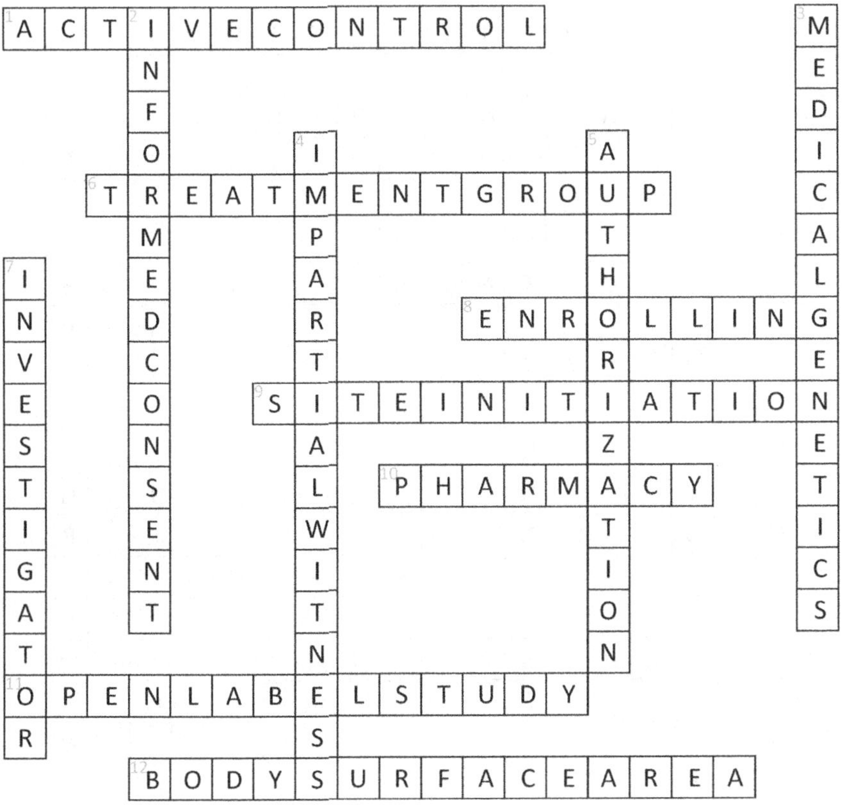

Across

1. ACTIVE CONTROL
6. TREATMENT GROUP
8. ENROLLING
9. SITE INITIATION
10. PHARMACY
11. OPEN LABEL STUDY
12. BODY SURFACE AREA

Down

2. INFORMED CONSENT
3. MEDICAL GENETICS
4. IMPARTIAL WITNESS
5. AUTHORIZATION
7. INVESTIGATOR

Crossword # 145

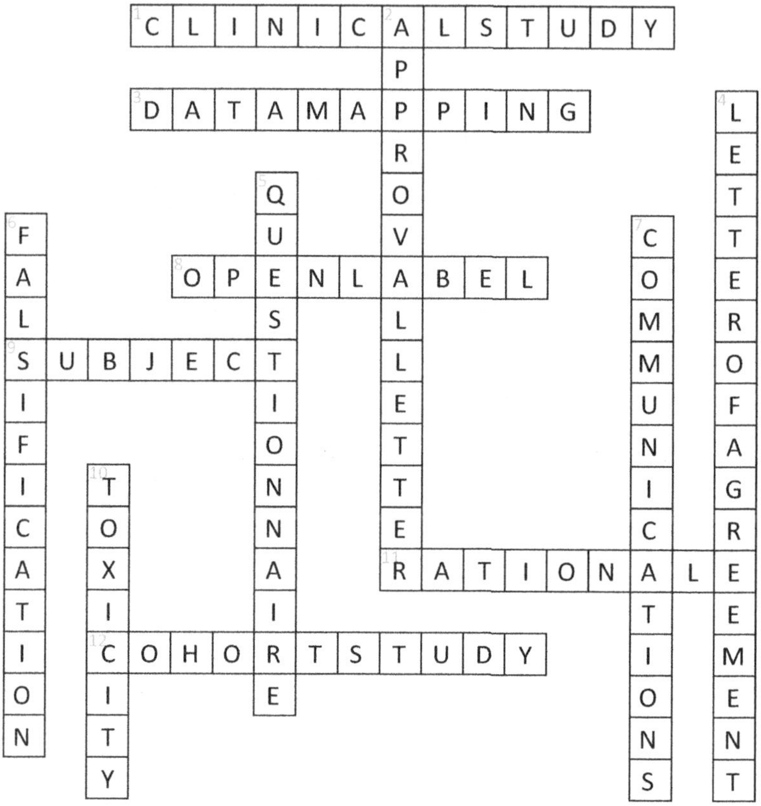

Across

1. CLINICAL STUDY
3. DATA MAPPING
8. OPEN LABEL
9. SUBJECT
11. RATIONALE
12. COHORT STUDY

Down

2. APPROVAL LETTER
4. LETTER OF AGREEMENT
5. QUESTIONNAIRE
6. FALSIFICATION
7. COMMUNICATIONS
10. TOXICITY

Crossword # 146

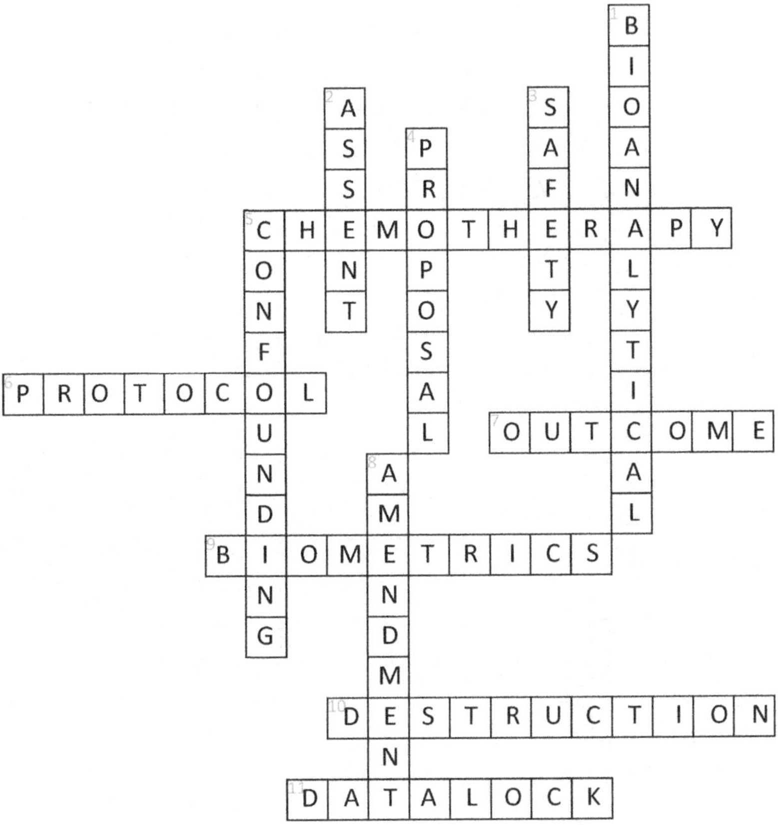

Across

5. CHEMOTHERAPY
6. PROTOCOL
7. OUTCOME
9. BIOMETRICS
10. DESTRUCTION
11. DATA LOCK

Down

1. BIO ANALYTICAL
2. ASSENT
3. SAFETY
4. PROPOSAL
5. CONFOUNDING
8. AMENDMENT

Crossword # 147

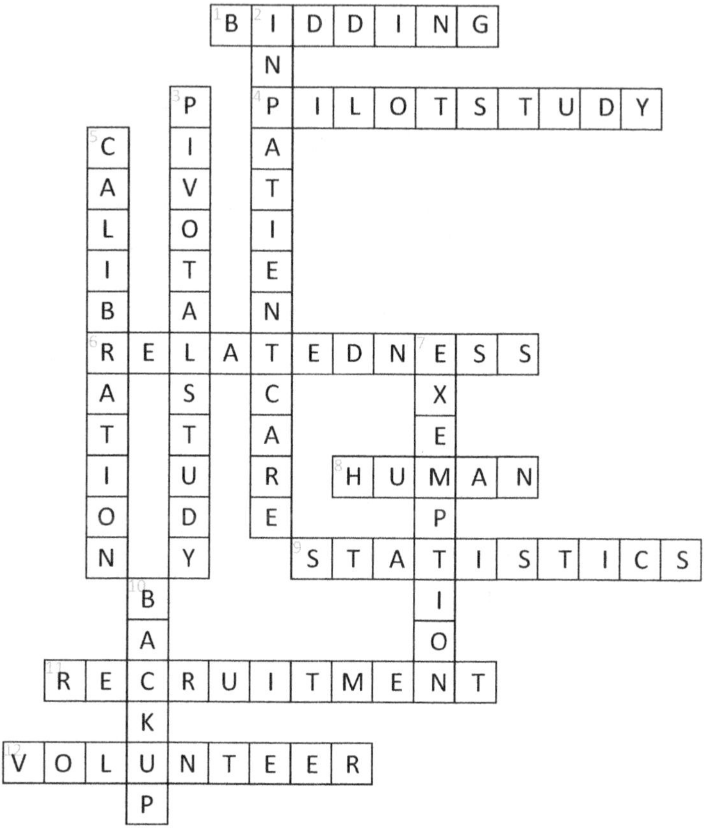

Across

1. BIDDING
4. PILOT STUDY
6. RELATEDNESS
8. HUMAN
9. STATISTICS
11. RECRUITMENT
12. VOLUNTEER

Down

2. INPATIENT CARE
3. PIVOTAL STUDY
5. CALIBRATION
7. EXEMPTION
10. BACKUP

Crossword # 148

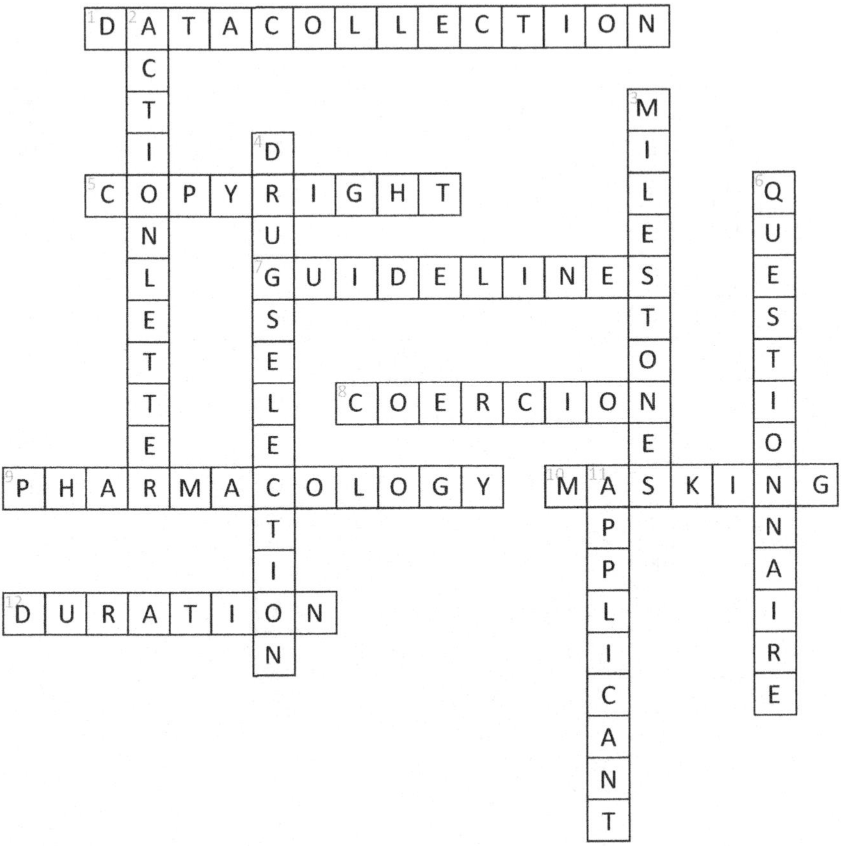

Across

1. DATA COLLECTION
5. COPYRIGHT
7. GUIDELINES
8. COERCION
9. PHARMACOLOGY
10. MASKING
12. DURATION

Down

2. ACTION LETTER
3. MILESTONES
4. DRUG SELECTION
6. QUESTIONNAIRE
11. APPLICANT

Crossword # 149

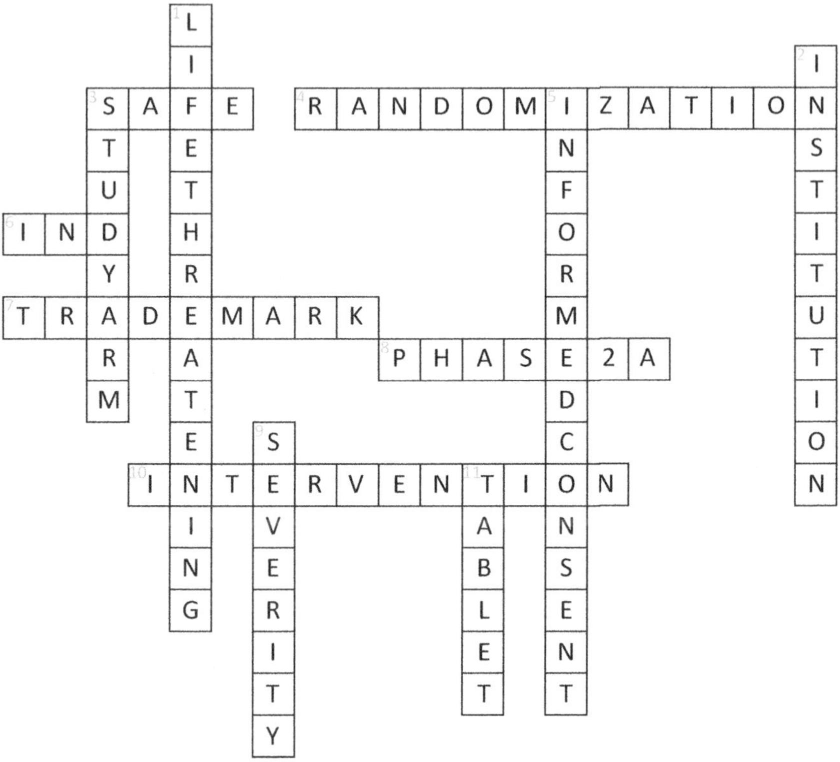

Across

3. SAFE
4. RANDOMIZATION
6. IND
7. TRADEMARK
8. PHASE 2A
10. INTERVENTION

Down

1. LIFE THREATENING
2. INSTITUTION
3. STUDY ARM
5. INFORMED CONSENT
9. SEVERITY
11. TABLET

IND: Investigational New Drug

Crossword # 150

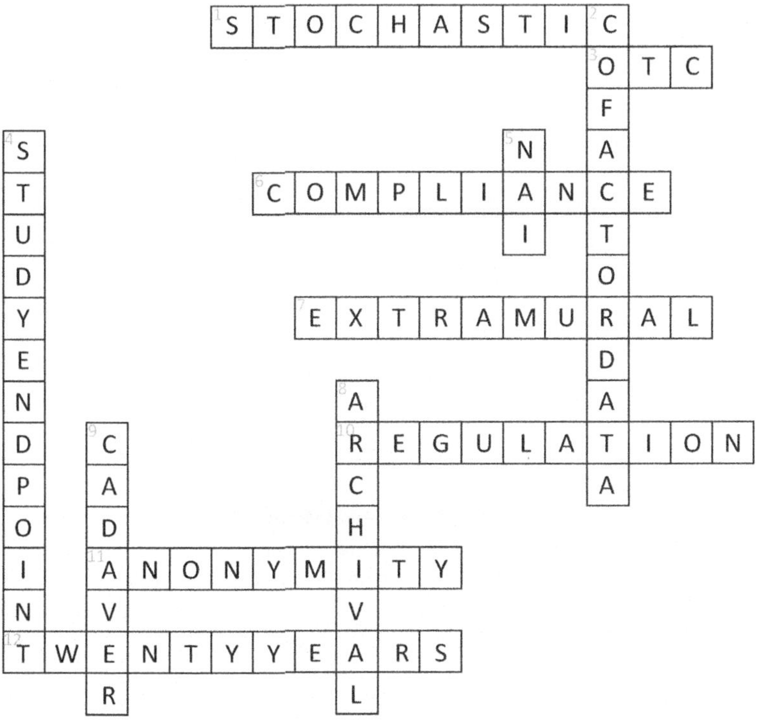

Across

1. STOCHASTIC
3. OTC
6. COMPLIANCE
7. EXTRAMURAL
10. REGULATION
11. ANONYMITY
12. TWENTY YEARS

Down

2. COFACTOR DATA
4. STUDY ENDPOINT
5. NAI
8. ARCHIVAL
9. CADAVER

OTC: Over The Counter; **NAI**: No Action Indicated

2

Keys for Jumbled Words

This section contains solution of 160 Jumbled Words.

Jumbled Words

1. SCBTAART

A	B	S	T	R	A	C	T

2. TCUCNIOLBAIYAT

A	C	C	O	U	N	T	A	B	I	L	I	T	Y

3. EARIDCCIATNOT

A	C	C	R	E	D	I	T	A	T	I	O	N

4. AEDDNMDU

A	D	D	E	N	D	U	M

5. DSAEVRE

A	D	V	E	R	S	E

6. AAGNED

A	G	E	N	D	A

7. MMNANEDTE

A	M	E	N	D	M	E	N	T

8. PLORVAPA

A	P	P	R	O	V	A	L

9. AVRAHCIL

A	R	C	H	I	V	A	L

10. STNAES

A	S	S	E	N	T

11. TUIDA

A	U	D	I	T

12. UASYTPO

A	U	T	O	P	S	Y

Jumbled Words

13. LESABIEN

B	A	S	E	L	I	N	E

14. SBAI

B	I	A	S

15. IALABITLOIYBIAV

B	I	O	A	V	A	I	L	A	B	I	L	I	T	Y

16. BIAIAVABELOL

B	I	O	A	V	A	I	L	A	B	L	E

17. BOCFNSAOMITRII

B	I	O	I	N	F	O	R	M	A	T	I	C	S

18. IOCRBITSME

B	I	O	M	E	T	R	I	C	S

19. POSNYSIS

S	Y	N	O	P	S	I	S

20. TIBIATOSSTSCI

B	I	O	S	T	A	T	I	S	T	I	C	S

21. LOCOETIGHBNOY

B	I	O	T	E	C	H	N	O	L	O	G	Y

22. NLDIB

B	L	I	N	D

23. LBGDNIIN

B	L	I	N	D	I	N	G

24. OTABCAILRNI

C	A	L	I	B	R	A	T	I	O	N

Jumbled Words

25. IERCNGIOACCN

C	A	R	C	I	N	O	G	E	N	I	C

26. CTSAAYULI

C	A	U	S	A	L	I	T	Y

27. IICCALNL

C	L	I	N	I	C	A	L

28. GDNOIC

C	O	D	I	N	G

29. OHCRTO

C	O	H	O	R	T

30. ORMROAATPC

C	O	M	P	A	R	A	T	O	R

31. AELCPOINMC

C	O	M	P	L	I	A	N	C	E

32. TIONACCOTMN

C	O	N	C	O	M	I	T	A	N	T

33. TIATIEDYNONCIFL

C	O	N	F	I	D	E	N	T	I	A	L	I	T	Y

34. OCTSNNE

C	O	N	S	E	N	T

35. RIIAAIONNOTTCNCD

C	O	N	T	R	A	I	N	D	I	C	A	T	I	O	N

36. CONORTL

C	O	N	T	R	O	L

Jumbled Words

37. CIATOORRLEN

C	O	R	R	E	L	A	T	I	O	N

38. SOVSCRROE

C	R	O	S	S	O	V	E	R

39. EADASATB

D	A	T	A	B	A	S	E

40. ODAEIITVN

D	E	V	I	A	T	I	O	N

41. CEIVDE

D	E	V	I	C	E

42. ISSDIGNAO

D	I	A	G	N	O	S	I	S

43. ESOCDYIRV

D	I	S	C	O	V	E	R	Y

44. SSEIADE

D	I	S	E	A	S	E

45. ENAUMDOOINTCT

D	O	C	U	M	E	N	T	A	T	I	O	N

46. DSOE

D	O	S	E

47. RTPODOU

D	R	O	P	O	U	T

48. URDG

D	R	U	G

Jumbled Words

49. FYEICFAC

E	F	F	I	C	A	C	Y

50. RIIALECPM

E	M	P	I	R	I	C	A	L

51. TIPENNDO

E	N	D	P	O	I	N	T

52. ODPYLEIIMGOE

E	P	I	D	E	M	I	O	L	O	G	Y

53. EISTCH

E	T	H	I	C	S

54. UXSEIOLCN

E	X	C	L	U	S	I	O	N

55. EELENAXIMRPT

E	X	P	E	R	I	M	E	N	T	A	L

56. FAD

F	D	A

57. TFLMIOANURO

F	O	R	M	U	L	A	T	I	O	N

58. ENGILEIUSD

G	U	I	D	E	L	I	N	E	S

59. HATSILOP

H	O	S	P	I	T	A	L

60. HSOEYTSHPI

H	Y	P	O	T	H	E	S	I	S

Jumbled Words

61. SNIUOICLN

I	N	C	L	U	S	I	O	N

62. TNNDIOIAIC

I	N	D	I	C	A	T	I	O	N

63. TCSENIPOIN

I	N	S	P	E	C	T	I	O	N

64. TICERATNONI

I	N	T	E	R	A	C	T	I	O	N

65. IENTTNOEIVRN

I	N	T	E	R	V	E	N	T	I	O	N

66. NEASIVVI

I	N	V	A	S	I	V	E

67. ETSGAIIVTONR

I	N	V	E	S	T	I	G	A	T	O	R

68. BLALE

L	A	B	E	L

69. YRORLABAOT

L	A	B	O	R	A	T	O	R	Y

70. LTCOISGIS

L	O	G	I	S	T	I	C	S

71. CURAMNSITP

M	A	N	U	S	C	R	I	P	T

72. EKMDAS

M	A	S	K	E	D

Jumbled Words

73. ENEDIIMC

M	E	D	I	C	I	N	E

74. MLASMBOEIT

M	E	T	A	B	O	L	I	S	M

75. NRMOGNIITO

M	O	N	I	T	O	R	I	N	G

76. AMORYTILT

M	O	R	T	A	L	I	T	Y

77. AEUTMGNCI

M	U	T	A	G	E	N	I	C

78. ERUMBNREG

N	U	R	E	M	B	E	R	G

79. OTERIBAVSALNO

O	B	S	E	R	V	A	T	I	O	N	A	L

80. LOTEURI

O	U	T	L	I	E	R

81. PENTTA

P	A	T	E	N	T

82. NIPATTE

P	A	T	I	E	N	T

83. TIPHSRCMAA

P	H	A	R	M	A	C	I	S	T

84. INASMAODCPHCMRAY

P	H	A	R	M	A	C	O	D	Y	N	A	M	I	C	S

Jumbled Words

85. EOCCINMPAOSMROHCA

P	H	A	R	M	A	C	O	E	C	O	N	O	M	I	C	S

86. AMPARKCTHCIISNEO

P	H	A	R	M	A	C	O	K	I	N	E	T	I	C	S

87. CHMPALOYAOGR

P	H	A	R	M	A	C	O	L	O	G	Y

88. LNACAVIEIPGHRMAOC

P	H	A	R	M	A	C	O	V	I	G	I	L	A	N	C	E

89. RPHAAMCY

P	H	A	R	M	A	C	Y

90. SPIHACNIY

P	H	Y	S	I	C	I	A	N

91. BEOPALC

P	L	A	C	E	B	O

92. PMGNRSOTKAIET

P	O	S	T	M	A	R	K	E	T	I	N	G

93. PTOYECN

P	O	T	E	N	C	Y

94. LRPCILENIAC

P	R	E	C	L	I	N	I	C	A	L

95. CIRPTNRPOSEI

P	R	E	S	C	R	I	P	T	I	O	N

96. ELVCRAEPEN

P	R	E	V	A	L	E	N	C	E

Jumbled Words

97. PECORJT

P	R	O	J	E	C	T

98. CIPROHATLCPY

P	R	O	P	H	Y	L	A	C	T	I	C

99. ARSLPPOO

P	R	O	P	O	S	A	L

100. PVPSETRICOE

P	R	O	S	P	E	C	T	I	V	E

101. OLOPCRTO

P	R	O	T	O	C	O	L

102. YAITUQL

Q	U	A	L	I	T	Y

103. QIRSEUINATEON

Q	U	E	S	T	I	O	N	N	A	I	R	E

104. MNRAOD

R	A	N	D	O	M

105. NRODMITANOAZI

R	A	N	D	O	M	I	Z	A	T	I	O	N

106. AOAINTRLE

R	A	T	I	O	N	A	L	E

107. CTEINMEURTR

R	E	C	R	U	I	T	M	E	N	T

108. SRRCEEEENF

R	E	F	E	R	E	N	C	E	S

Jumbled Words

109. MEGNRIE

R	E	G	I	M	E	N

110. ITENUROGLA

R	E	G	U	L	A	T	I	O	N

111. GYOULTRERA

R	E	G	U	L	A	T	O	R	Y

112. RRTPEO

R	E	P	O	R	T

113. RAESEHRC

R	E	S	E	A	R	C	H

114. EVSECRTETOPIR

R	E	T	R	O	S	P	E	C	T	I	V	E

115. TSFAEY

S	A	F	E	T	Y

116. CERINGSNE

S	C	R	E	E	N	I	N	G

117. SOERCU

S	O	U	R	C	E

118. ICSTISNAIATT

S	T	A	T	I	S	T	I	C	I	A	N

119. UTJBCSE

S	U	B	J	E	C	T

120. SEEPSURDE

S	U	P	E	R	S	E	D	E

Jumbled Words

121. ETPELAMT

T	E	M	P	L	A	T	E

122. OTTREEIAGCN

T	E	R	A	T	O	G	E	N	I	C

123. PAYRTEH

T	H	E	R	A	P	Y

124. XIICTYTO

T	O	X	I	C	I	T	Y

125. RNSOILANTTA

T	R	A	N	S	L	A	T	I	O	N

126. TTANMRETE

T	R	E	A	T	M	E	N	T

127. ILRAT

T	R	I	A	L

128. IBNUNIGNLD

U	N	B	L	I	N	D	I	N	G

129. VLITDIAONA

V	A	L	I	D	A	T	I	O	N

130. SEIRVON

V	E	R	S	I	O	N

131. RLTOUNAYV

V	O	L	U	N	T	A	R	Y

132. NRUOLETEV

V	O	L	U	N	T	E	E	R

Jumbled Words

133. LEURLEBAVN

V	U	L	N	E	R	A	B	L	E

134. OLBMTEN

B	E	L	M	O	N	T

135. BAIS

B	I	A	S

136. YTAIAUSCL

C	A	U	S	A	L	I	T	Y

137. RRAIOODTCNO

C	O	O	R	D	I	N	A	T	O	R

138. ROTPONIEAS

O	P	E	R	A	T	I	O	N	S

139. YTACSALT

C	A	T	A	L	Y	S	T

140. OCRTNTAC

C	O	N	T	R	A	C	T

141. DEOGAS

D	O	S	A	G	E

142. RARTEAUMLX

E	X	T	R	A	M	U	R	A	L

143. NBCAOATRIFI

F	A	B	R	I	C	A	T	I	O	N

144. GRTNA

G	R	A	N	T

Jumbled Words

145. EMAIFDNNIIINOTC

I	N	D	E	M	N	I	F	I	C	A	T	I	O	N

146. TSCOCIMNUD

M	I	S	C	O	N	D	U	C	T

147. KSRI

R	I	S	K

148. OMPSTMY

S	Y	M	P	T	O	M

149. YRSVEU

S	U	R	V	E	Y

150. TIWSENS

W	I	T	N	E	S	S

151. LCINEUETRTM

M	U	L	T	I	C	E	N	T	E	R

152. HESPA

P	H	A	S	E

153. OSRNSEEP

R	E	S	P	O	N	S	E

154. TESAG

S	T	A	G	E

155. LROONTC

C	O	N	T	R	O	L

156. TDTASAE

D	A	T	A	S	E	T

Jumbled Words

157. NIPDAERCCSY

D	I	S	C	R	E	P	A	N	C	Y

158. RLELON

E	N	R	O	L	L

159. EROYLPXATRO

E	X	P	L	O	R	A	T	O	R	Y

160. LTPAIAMIR

I	M	P	A	R	T	I	A	L

3

Keys for Word Search

This section contains solution of 31 exercises containing 10 words each pertaining to a particular clinical trial element/activity/process. For the ease of readers solutions and abbreviations have been elaborated at the bottom of the table.

Word Search

1. Clinical Project Milestones (i)

J	N	B	K	P	E	W	R	X	Z	K	J	T	K	C	S	Z	Q	F	E
K	U	Q	P	R	Z	J	F	M	S	T	E	D	U	H	K	W	Z	L	Z
V	Q	M	H	O	U	B	A	C	K	K	R	K	A	P	P	A	A	R	V
N	W	V	N	J	U	V	X	O	Z	Y	N	A	U	U	N	V	Y	G	W
I	K	K	P	E	J	U	J	K	A	B	P	T	D	E	O	R	M	R	O
P	F	I	K	C	J	M	D	U	Q	K	E	R	C	R	Z	N	N	U	U
P	A	Q	A	T	D	V	P	T	X	S	E	T	P	O	V	G	D	L	O
R	W	I	D	P	C	H	K	X	E	L	O	P	R	W	T	A	H	D	O
O	S	M	H	L	T	S	B	S	A	C	A	I	A	A	Y	X	K	H	S
C	D	G	K	A	M	C	A	D	N	Y	L	W	T	T	I	P	Q	G	P
U	M	V	O	N	X	B	T	K	R	A	D	T	I	H	I	N	K	Y	F
R	N	B	E	M	A	C	G	O	R	I	V	L	Z	D	I	M	I	I	P
E	J	C	F	T	P	L	T	A	T	T	I	M	T	V	F	W	D	N	V
M	Y	N	A	T	Z	A	I	V	A	B	L	R	Q	Z	S	C	J	P	G
E	Z	D	H	R	L	V	Y	X	I	Q	Z	Z	R	G	F	I	S	D	H
N	R	Y	U	U	O	F	C	S	W	G	Z	W	R	S	O	U	V	B	R
T	D	S	G	J	I	R	A	I	M	A	F	Z	R	O	D	H	P	O	D
W	M	E	F	C	T	E	F	W	E	C	A	P	P	R	O	V	A	L	S
K	R	V	X	G	F	S	I	T	E	S	E	L	E	C	T	I	O	N	B
T	I	E	J	N	E	S	T	W	N	R	J	U	Y	X	A	Y	S	B	R

IP (Investigational Product) Procurement, Project Plan, Database Set-up, Regulatory Approval, Feasibility, Training, FPV (First Patient Visit), SIV (Site Initiation Visit), EC (Ethics Committee) Approval, Site Selection

Word Search

2. Clinical Project Milestones (ii)

L	I	Q	I	X	J	S	W	L	F	U	P	Z	T	B	R	L	V	I	Y
M	N	X	F	E	A	A	V	E	F	Y	W	B	T	T	T	Q	H	N	Z
D	Z	Q	P	R	L	S	A	X	H	E	B	Y	V	N	R	Z	M	T	C
A	M	B	N	O	K	F	Z	R	F	N	Z	P	E	O	P	F	V	E	F
T	T	H	T	T	I	A	M	N	C	E	L	M	D	K	D	U	F	R	Q
A	K	F	H	B	G	R	F	G	N	H	E	I	K	K	A	F	Y	I	D
L	Q	A	C	V	S	M	L	B	W	G	I	Z	S	W	P	U	F	M	Z
O	R	U	K	C	M	F	W	F	A	T	C	V	D	F	U	N	I	A	G
C	B	O	H	N	I	F	Y	N	E	H	N	O	A	V	B	D	U	N	T
K	Z	K	K	Y	P	G	A	P	B	D	L	L	X	L	L	R	F	A	T
E	O	X	A	D	J	M	L	Q	B	Z	V	Z	Z	T	I	F	T	L	T
H	D	N	F	W	A	J	X	U	N	C	U	C	B	E	C	Z	V	Y	Y
S	D	S	I	T	E	C	L	O	S	E	O	U	T	N	A	C	G	S	L
K	P	C	A	Q	H	T	P	E	V	M	R	F	A	E	T	T	R	I	C
N	Z	D	X	Y	A	O	M	B	B	W	W	H	L	S	I	W	M	S	Z
O	W	R	H	C	L	E	X	U	U	X	I	N	Z	C	O	H	U	G	L
L	D	H	U	W	T	R	I	A	L	C	L	O	S	E	N	U	A	C	N
W	M	T	V	L	P	N	K	H	D	O	X	L	I	R	N	R	I	B	E

Data Lock, CSR (Clinical Study Report), Archival, Data Management, LPV (Last Patient Visit), LPET (Last Patient Enter Treatment), Site Close-out, Trial Close, Publication, Interim Analysis

Word Search

3. Ethics Committee

H	U	N	N	A	U	S	O	A	P	P	R	O	V	A	L	N	R	H	I
G	B	O	B	Z	S	O	A	Q	G	V	P	Q	A	S	Z	I	Z	N	H
X	B	D	C	O	K	F	D	W	T	K	Y	W	N	T	P	X	E	F	D
E	W	X	U	W	L	Q	J	H	A	V	E	W	W	Z	B	A	N	V	G
Q	I	N	I	T	I	A	L	R	E	V	I	E	W	K	F	K	L	Y	D
I	Q	F	Q	G	Y	T	L	V	H	M	N	J	U	F	H	T	A	Q	M
J	F	S	X	J	X	M	L	P	I	S	Z	A	H	E	C	U	Z	V	C
U	F	A	V	O	R	A	B	L	E	O	P	I	N	I	O	N	U	K	D
T	F	D	I	S	A	P	P	R	O	V	A	L	R	T	T	O	E	T	Y
X	H	L	W	Z	X	M	F	N	W	V	H	R	D	B	F	Q	I	U	Z
I	W	W	M	F	Y	P	D	Q	Q	P	M	P	O	S	M	S	V	E	I
C	K	X	E	D	V	T	T	B	J	V	D	T	R	C	E	I	F	I	C
A	Z	C	V	X	E	X	P	E	D	I	T	E	D	R	E	V	I	E	W
R	B	V	R	X	Z	N	C	X	Z	U	B	V	I	M	N	F	W	G	G
Q	U	O	R	U	M	Y	E	D	X	M	C	H	S	K	G	U	Z	D	X
N	Y	I	K	X	U	A	F	G	E	Y	U	P	M	B	X	K	E	B	H
D	C	P	S	S	O	D	Y	M	A	X	Z	Y	C	Q	E	J	H	R	B
A	R	O	K	W	N	X	A	J	R	L	O	X	W	C	Y	P	V	Z	V

Approval, Initial Review, EC (Ethics Committee), Favorable Opinion, Disapproval, IRB (Institutional Review Board), IEC (Independent Ethics Committee), Expedited Review, Quorum, Members

Word Search

4. Investigational Product

E	Y	G	S	S	Z	K	N	U	M	G	K	M	D	S	Q	J	B	R	K
C	O	A	Y	J	S	Y	F	N	O	I	G	G	Z	G	D	P	G	G	U
D	X	N	H	E	H	S	J	M	T	H	W	I	N	M	Y	H	A	N	J
E	A	L	B	N	Z	N	H	N	E	Y	O	I	Z	P	O	X	H	N	G
S	G	R	O	S	R	I	Q	I	M	C	S	Y	K	H	R	A	Q	A	R
T	M	J	M	U	Q	T	K	M	P	N	G	A	D	X	G	A	B	C	E
R	I	V	T	X	Y	D	K	X	E	M	I	U	J	E	V	E	Q	C	C
U	A	E	Z	B	M	S	H	P	R	F	E	S	K	R	C	Y	U	O	E
C	R	Q	S	L	N	H	S	P	A	O	X	N	X	Q	S	O	K	U	I
T	B	X	T	O	S	I	J	N	T	B	R	Q	T	Z	X	C	E	N	P
I	U	S	O	X	D	B	U	W	U	T	D	C	I	X	H	R	X	T	T
O	I	D	R	A	Y	Z	J	J	R	H	S	Q	H	W	G	B	P	A	Q
N	Y	V	A	E	B	F	V	D	E	R	Y	E	R	N	O	T	U	B	S
M	V	U	G	R	N	K	D	U	L	M	R	U	O	M	P	D	V	I	U
G	V	U	E	Z	E	V	W	S	O	L	X	J	N	V	J	A	Y	L	Z
L	D	J	Z	W	D	I	F	R	G	U	W	B	W	I	X	Z	D	I	Z
U	X	D	X	Z	U	Z	V	H	T	F	R	G	Q	M	Z	H	L	T	Q
K	G	A	R	W	A	C	C	E	S	S	C	O	N	T	R	O	L	Y	I

COA (Certificate of Analysis), Destruction, Return, Storage, Shipment, Dispensing, Temperature Log, Access Control, Accountability, Receipt

Word Search

5. Clinical Trial Monitoring

M	I	M	H	H	B	S	A	E	R	E	V	I	E	W	M	P	I	T	D
O	Y	P	F	W	J	R	X	J	Y	S	Z	H	F	Q	L	U	P	J	X
N	O	R	R	X	N	D	Z	Y	J	C	R	F	R	E	V	I	E	W	I
I	N	D	L	O	M	O	F	A	W	X	A	G	H	M	Y	N	B	F	A
T	T	G	S	A	T	U	C	R	H	G	I	X	S	V	D	A	H	E	D
O	F	X	C	K	U	O	T	Y	U	L	O	W	C	G	W	J	A	R	E
R	N	Z	N	V	I	P	C	S	I	N	A	D	W	X	K	S	S	X	V
I	A	S	D	W	I	H	G	O	M	A	F	R	U	D	Z	V	A	C	I
N	V	S	A	C	R	F	C	O	L	L	E	C	T	I	O	N	Y	Q	A
G	H	S	T	P	O	V	N	A	Y	C	C	H	D	F	Q	E	H	H	T
R	Y	V	F	I	T	R	S	B	K	P	O	I	T	I	O	J	G	B	I
E	D	I	T	B	T	N	T	S	I	B	T	M	L	W	D	R	R	O	O
P	S	L	A	Q	P	D	C	J	V	X	Z	H	P	N	A	U	G	V	N
O	G	S	D	C	Q	V	Z	A	P	N	Q	V	T	L	O	C	Q	F	S
R	E	G	U	L	A	T	O	R	Y	C	O	M	P	L	I	A	N	C	E
T	C	O	R	I	A	E	X	Z	G	C	E	F	N	D	D	A	C	H	Z
M	I	P	A	C	C	O	U	N	T	A	B	I	L	I	T	Y	N	R	E
F	Z	Y	F	K	O	H	N	L	M	C	V	K	V	W	F	E	Z	C	L
E	O	J	Y	H	J	Y	I	C	D	R	E	V	I	E	W	Z	W	L	E

Monitoring Report, SDV (Source Data Verification), Protocol Compliance, Deviations, SAE (Serious Adverse Event) Review, CRF (Case Report Form) Review, CRF Collection, Regulatory Compliance, IP (Investigational Product) Accountability, ICD (Informed Consent Document) Review

Word Search

6. ICH-GCP Required Elements for ICD (i)

R	Y	I	W	Y	A	L	C	O	M	P	E	N	S	A	T	I	O	N	S
S	A	Q	L	X	E	C	L	B	G	U	J	A	C	F	C	A	P	T	L
T	Z	L	E	O	N	B	G	J	V	X	T	Y	B	S	S	G	I	T	S
U	E	F	T	K	P	A	W	B	P	K	B	M	T	L	R	F	G	R	F
D	U	O	W	E	G	R	P	U	R	P	O	S	E	Q	E	G	I	I	C
Y	M	R	G	S	R	D	O	M	L	V	U	Q	Q	N	X	F	B	A	Z
P	F	E	D	Y	R	N	O	R	S	N	S	P	E	O	A	K	Y	L	J
R	Z	S	Y	D	Q	L	A	E	A	S	X	B	Y	A	P	L	L	T	D
O	O	E	P	F	E	E	Y	T	S	T	D	T	L	U	K	K	A	R	U
C	G	E	Y	P	C	D	R	D	I	E	E	H	J	S	F	Y	F	E	X
E	F	A	O	U	Q	C	C	Q	T	V	X	D	R	J	R	X	X	A	K
D	W	B	D	X	X	Z	D	C	A	K	E	C	P	A	Z	W	Z	T	L
U	A	L	L	E	X	P	E	N	S	E	S	C	T	A	I	T	V	M	C
R	H	E	B	M	J	P	I	Y	Q	F	B	N	O	D	Y	W	U	E	I
E	H	R	K	F	X	H	K	A	P	M	U	F	N	U	L	M	A	N	K
O	P	I	N	E	K	U	T	Q	Y	L	W	O	U	N	R	D	E	T	Z
V	B	S	C	N	P	L	V	A	O	M	T	S	D	C	O	S	L	N	V
Q	I	K	X	T	M	W	C	V	K	Q	L	W	B	O	Z	M	E	C	T
Q	S	S	Q	G	A	D	K	G	E	C	J	W	B	D	P	F	G	G	H

Study Procedure, Foreseeable Risks, Compensation, Purpose, Expenses, Alternative Course, Prorated Payment, Expected Benefits, Voluntary, Trial Treatment

Word Search

7. ICH-GCP Required Elements for ICD (ii)

S	E	G	N	N	T	T	R	B	Y	W	V	K	Z	B	P	X	A	T	L
F	M	T	R	E	S	E	A	R	C	H	S	T	U	D	Y	S	C	X	Q
E	E	D	A	O	N	V	I	F	C	P	P	U	W	H	T	E	X	R	A
R	R	J	R	R	B	A	S	K	Z	Y	R	B	C	C	P	A	F	A	N
I	G	C	E	V	Z	S	L	T	B	R	J	A	E	S	K	L	T	N	V
G	E	R	O	Z	I	K	L	G	O	U	H	J	A	N	K	V	O	D	Q
H	N	U	W	N	S	Z	B	E	B	V	B	L	R	X	I	J	V	O	R
T	C	V	N	J	F	M	V	G	V	U	A	P	S	D	H	T	I	M	M
T	Y	B	Y	R	Y	I	P	B	S	T	P	U	Q	X	W	R	R	A	M
O	C	T	Q	A	K	E	D	F	N	Q	D	Q	Z	S	D	Z	J	L	J
R	O	I	I	K	U	B	O	E	L	K	K	Y	R	A	J	F	Q	L	Z
E	N	J	V	S	T	R	M	K	N	E	D	F	T	T	H	R	I	O	I
F	T	J	O	C	E	I	C	Z	M	T	S	U	I	C	J	J	T	C	I
U	A	P	W	B	R	J	N	K	B	G	I	T	R	D	Q	J	K	A	M
S	C	A	M	E	A	T	Z	B	X	D	R	A	I	A	O	D	B	T	D
E	T	U	P	X	S	R	C	A	E	E	C	T	L	P	T	F	N	I	N
Y	N	X	A	R	J	J	R	S	S	T	K	D	W	I	C	I	U	O	O
V	E	I	J	T	E	R	M	I	N	A	T	I	O	N	T	S	O	N	Y
R	E	S	P	O	N	S	I	B	I	L	I	T	I	E	S	Y	X	N	G

Right to Refuse, Emergency Contact, Research Study, Termination, Responsibilities, Confidentiality, Duration, Random Allocation, Number of Subjects, Experimental Aspect

Word Search

8. Clinical Trial Stakeholders

A	D	R	D	K	Y	U	H	S	S	Y	E	A	I	T	Q	K	I	I	S
K	R	R	E	L	Z	D	T	L	P	E	J	D	S	P	R	J	N	Y	M
H	U	A	X	G	C	B	M	I	H	V	Y	C	P	R	Y	G	V	F	O
N	F	Y	V	J	U	S	U	K	G	M	N	E	O	I	P	C	E	F	S
T	T	Y	R	F	P	L	T	K	Q	M	I	T	N	W	S	N	S	K	U
V	E	P	E	T	O	W	A	U	H	Z	I	C	S	M	I	P	T	L	S
N	E	D	C	K	X	V	G	T	D	N	N	P	O	T	Q	E	I	J	G
P	J	D	M	R	O	D	G	F	O	Y	N	Z	R	A	R	N	G	L	K
H	K	Q	F	U	B	J	F	M	C	R	S	X	W	S	J	L	A	M	X
Z	T	P	H	V	O	Y	Y	C	A	M	Y	U	P	P	I	Y	T	L	D
Q	S	O	E	R	N	D	N	W	I	U	J	A	B	G	I	I	O	Z	O
K	G	A	O	V	U	H	I	C	W	F	I	D	G	J	Z	T	R	Q	K
K	D	V	D	T	R	X	R	B	Q	P	I	Y	D	E	E	X	N	G	B
K	C	U	S	T	F	O	Z	W	M	K	E	M	L	H	N	C	F	P	G
K	W	R	O	H	T	X	M	F	A	E	H	X	M	M	R	C	T	Q	B
A	S	U	B	I	N	V	E	S	T	I	G	A	T	O	R	T	Y	S	J
I	T	N	D	G	F	K	H	Y	M	N	Y	I	B	H	J	E	I	I	T
S	C	U	Q	N	I	C	R	O	D	H	R	T	B	S	F	J	Y	R	Y
J	A	K	T	F	C	M	D	G	W	A	O	F	I	K	P	R	O	B	Z

Regulatory Agency, Study Subjects, Study Monitor, Auditor, Sub Investigator, CRO (Contract Research Organization), Sponsor, Investigator, SMO (Site Management Organization), IRB (Institutional Review Board)

Word Search

9. Sponsor's Responsibilities (i)

Y	A	O	M	D	X	I	P	M	A	N	A	G	E	M	E	N	T	M	N
W	B	W	Y	Y	D	Z	N	O	V	T	V	I	F	T	X	I	I	O	P
J	K	B	N	B	Q	A	H	D	O	Z	P	D	N	B	T	P	I	X	O
R	S	Z	S	X	I	X	T	R	K	B	T	E	M	U	K	T	S	L	C
B	R	S	A	I	U	K	W	A	O	F	M	E	S	O	C	W	W	D	R
Q	I	L	R	R	R	I	H	D	M	P	U	S	P	E	W	Q	N	Q	A
L	B	J	R	X	F	B	T	T	O	A	A	K	L	O	V	A	M	X	G
H	X	E	X	O	U	S	E	L	Q	F	N	E	Z	V	N	O	Y	T	R
M	J	X	G	U	H	H	E	H	H	I	S	A	R	J	N	T	N	A	E
M	K	B	W	V	Q	V	C	L	B	E	I	P	G	S	M	A	E	L	E
I	L	S	D	D	E	N	S	F	T	M	J	W	H	E	A	E	D	D	M
L	B	A	S	D	M	H	V	I	D	C	D	J	J	K	M	I	L	N	E
K	H	R	D	E	X	F	S	S	V	G	F	P	A	D	G	E	D	R	N
B	G	C	L	K	A	T	R	I	A	L	P	L	A	N	N	I	N	G	T
O	I	S	T	I	F	O	X	K	W	E	U	U	E	V	E	T	Z	T	S
P	R	O	T	O	C	O	L	D	E	V	E	L	O	P	M	E	N	T	F
B	R	Q	H	K	P	U	B	L	I	C	A	T	I	O	N	D	M	W	T
T	M	T	R	I	A	L	M	A	N	A	G	E	M	E	N	T	T	O	O
Z	R	E	G	U	L	A	T	O	R	Y	A	P	P	R	O	V	A	L	Q

IP (Investigational Product) Management, Trial Planning, Protocol Development, Publication, Trial Management, Regulatory Approval, ICD (Informed Consent Document) Development, Site Selection, Data Management, Agreements

Word Search

10. Sponsor's Responsibilities (ii)

D	C	R	F	D	E	V	E	L	O	P	M	E	N	T	U	S	M	G	Q
N	C	V	A	I	L	T	A	B	S	H	Q	E	U	G	H	S	N	C	J
P	O	J	S	Y	L	G	O	Y	A	J	F	L	G	L	T	I	M	Y	W
V	M	Q	G	I	X	Q	L	D	F	N	Z	X	O	F	T	P	I	E	K
P	G	Z	V	M	R	B	S	I	E	U	T	E	J	I	A	P	Q	V	L
B	A	X	N	V	C	Y	H	L	T	H	I	K	D	M	O	F	Z	K	N
X	P	Y	I	L	N	K	I	S	Y	Z	R	U	M	K	I	X	Y	V	R
G	L	C	M	L	B	E	D	E	R	R	A	E	S	I	A	W	Q	X	P
W	T	C	T	E	L	O	S	H	E	R	R	Z	E	B	H	W	H	X	F
B	R	J	Y	O	N	C	S	R	P	R	E	P	A	R	A	T	I	O	N
P	B	C	F	Z	V	T	R	E	O	H	L	N	C	M	U	T	C	Y	R
J	R	B	T	M	H	Q	S	P	R	X	H	W	N	O	F	H	R	S	C
I	N	V	E	S	T	I	G	A	T	O	R	T	R	A	I	N	I	N	G
J	E	A	H	P	Y	V	K	N	I	Z	P	M	K	X	B	H	G	S	R
Q	J	N	T	F	U	W	M	O	N	I	T	O	R	I	N	G	B	F	R
O	A	R	E	M	P	D	Y	E	G	D	A	S	D	N	M	E	H	E	R
G	P	E	R	I	O	D	I	C	R	E	P	O	R	T	I	N	G	J	S
P	O	I	B	D	E	V	E	L	O	P	M	E	N	T	Q	K	I	S	L
T	G	C	P	C	O	M	P	L	I	A	N	C	E	J	N	L	W	Q	U

CRF (Case Report Form) Development, Auditing, Payments, Safety Reporting, CSR (Clinical Study Report) Preparation, Investigator Training, Monitoring, Periodic Reporting, IB Development, GCP (Good Clinical Practice) Compliance

Word Search

11. Investigator's Responsibilities (i)

Q	D	T	K	R	A	D	S	H	M	J	M	W	X	F	Y	Z	E	J	R
I	A	G	O	U	I	P	A	B	P	T	W	D	V	I	E	C	S	Y	G
C	T	C	S	H	D	C	F	R	X	M	M	X	D	Y	N	H	O	P	C
D	A	P	E	Y	R	B	E	E	B	G	F	J	B	E	K	T	U	E	Z
A	C	C	P	O	T	M	T	C	Z	M	R	I	D	S	J	G	R	R	O
D	O	O	N	I	V	Q	Y	O	B	O	B	N	S	M	A	J	C	I	I
M	L	M	A	K	E	I	R	R	Q	N	O	O	P	Y	O	G	E	O	P
I	L	P	K	U	Z	Z	E	D	Q	P	D	H	S	Z	D	P	D	D	M
N	E	L	N	M	B	K	P	R	S	S	P	S	Y	W	Y	I	O	I	A
I	C	I	F	M	C	E	O	E	S	B	L	G	K	N	O	T	C	C	N
S	T	A	F	M	R	G	R	T	C	N	U	B	Z	D	I	Q	U	R	A
T	I	N	C	V	U	R	T	E	U	M	A	K	U	N	I	N	M	E	G
R	O	C	U	O	O	A	I	N	X	V	T	K	N	K	L	G	E	P	E
A	N	E	Z	C	Q	N	N	T	Y	E	K	R	I	L	J	O	N	O	M
T	Z	U	B	G	M	Y	G	I	B	K	C	P	S	B	H	T	T	R	E
I	B	R	N	V	N	N	S	O	U	T	O	E	M	J	P	S	A	T	N
O	I	M	P	N	J	Q	L	N	T	W	V	Z	H	C	R	M	T	I	T
N	V	N	N	M	E	D	I	C	A	L	C	A	R	E	I	O	I	N	L
E	U	X	T	Y	N	X	V	X	B	Z	G	H	G	S	Y	Y	O	G	A
S	M	K	C	W	I	Q	E	J	L	P	I	I	M	O	X	F	N	S	I

ICD (Informed Consent Document) Administration, Data Collection, GCP (Good Clinical Practice) Compliance, Safety Reporting, Record Retention, IRB (Institutional Review Board) Correspondence, Medical Care, Source Documentation, Periodic Reportings, IP Management

Word Search

12. Investigator's Responsibilities (ii)

K	V	Q	E	E	Y	G	U	W	Z	J	T	I	Z	J	A	Q	T	E	A
S	P	A	T	I	E	N	T	C	O	U	N	S	E	L	I	N	G	S	C
R	W	G	V	V	T	E	W	N	L	G	W	B	I	V	V	J	E	Q	C
V	J	R	D	K	R	W	I	O	L	Q	G	Z	F	F	Z	I	I	W	E
T	M	E	O	B	T	Q	V	L	S	I	G	Q	I	N	T	A	E	V	S
D	O	E	M	F	S	Z	R	U	S	E	U	L	Q	U	L	Y	Q	D	S
A	X	M	M	B	S	L	Q	I	P	H	H	A	D	Q	I	E	P	C	C
D	A	E	X	E	X	K	E	N	O	Q	C	F	L	N	J	Z	F	F	O
W	F	N	A	K	C	D	M	A	U	U	O	A	D	D	E	G	G	R	N
D	Q	T	B	D	N	H	C	L	U	N	V	P	Z	G	I	M	J	E	T
Z	J	S	Q	Z	D	X	R	B	O	I	R	N	I	V	J	B	X	S	R
U	C	L	Z	D	S	X	F	I	H	L	J	X	D	R	S	C	T	O	O
H	H	R	R	E	B	O	T	C	S	J	L	M	K	I	O	P	N	L	L
T	E	S	Z	E	O	A	R	H	V	U	T	H	V	R	M	S	Y	U	F
N	K	E	P	E	C	A	P	X	H	Y	S	I	Z	A	K	T	U	T	E
A	M	W	R	O	C	R	F	C	O	M	P	L	E	T	I	O	N	I	D
I	N	Q	L	Z	A	D	R	M	A	N	A	G	E	M	E	N	T	O	S
C	M	L	V	R	H	A	K	X	L	O	B	Z	V	I	B	L	Z	N	O
T	A	P	R	O	T	O	C	O	L	C	O	M	P	L	I	A	N	C	E
C	O	N	F	I	D	E	N	T	I	A	L	I	T	Y	J	M	Z	M	F

Patient Counseling, Agreements, Allocation of Duties, Archival, Access Control, DCF (Data Clarification Form) Resolution, CRF (Case Report Form) Completion, ADR (Adverse Drug Reaction) Management, Protocol Compliance, Confidentiality

Word Search

13. IRB Responsibilities

D	R	G	W	A	B	X	N	X	H	F	D	H	Y	E	B	J	W	D	B
A	P	E	F	A	R	N	I	Z	T	R	C	W	M	F	C	F	R	O	R
G	R	I	V	M	C	O	M	P	O	S	I	T	I	O	N	I	I	N	L
Y	V	G	M	I	X	V	V	D	Z	C	V	R	C	W	R	S	T	X	R
Z	E	C	S	N	E	L	A	V	V	Q	V	U	Q	T	L	C	T	W	E
T	X	P	L	U	C	W	J	N	M	J	A	B	Z	Q	T	Q	E	G	C
R	P	C	M	T	J	V	O	F	W	O	M	L	O	O	O	I	N	J	O
I	E	O	B	E	O	I	Y	F	R	T	L	C	B	N	V	R	P	I	R
A	D	M	Q	S	J	W	B	L	D	V	G	U	I	E	S	H	R	N	D
L	I	P	G	O	K	S	O	E	F	O	C	I	R	K	W	J	O	I	R
A	T	L	W	F	Y	O	L	K	Z	D	C	G	G	P	Z	F	C	T	E
P	E	I	B	M	S	N	M	N	X	R	N	U	F	U	M	O	E	I	T
P	D	A	N	E	S	L	U	Q	C	I	A	Q	M	R	R	O	D	A	E
R	R	N	L	E	I	U	V	R	U	K	L	Y	R	E	E	K	U	L	N
O	E	C	U	T	U	E	O	N	B	X	D	F	P	P	N	U	R	R	T
V	V	E	M	I	V	J	I	L	M	E	Z	Y	L	M	W	T	E	E	I
A	I	X	V	N	T	T	A	Y	Q	D	U	P	W	H	V	F	S	V	O
L	E	B	N	G	N	Y	K	Y	V	X	O	O	D	Q	V	E	D	I	N
B	W	R	R	O	T	O	N	K	E	M	Q	K	Y	Z	A	E	L	E	A
H	A	I	C	H	B	M	K	A	C	T	Q	W	G	Z	H	D	V	W	H

Trial Approval, Expedited Review, GCP (Good Clinical Practice) Compliance, Minutes of Meeting, Written Procedures, Composition, Initial Review, Record Retention, Review of Documents, Continuing Review

Word Search

14. Documents Required for Initial IRB Review

M	M	A	S	G	C	J	T	Z	K	K	E	B	N	Q	J	O	D	B	T
K	E	D	Y	A	V	L	Z	Q	G	S	I	Z	L	V	L	C	F	S	E
D	S	V	V	K	F	K	O	F	D	X	E	R	G	Q	I	T	Q	O	I
Z	U	E	R	N	U	E	F	T	B	B	A	Y	L	A	N	I	G	O	S
S	W	R	K	V	V	L	T	F	X	T	M	N	K	E	O	P	H	B	X
M	Q	T	K	P	S	K	H	Y	S	I	O	G	M	B	J	N	Q	H	S
I	Z	I	B	Y	U	M	B	V	I	H	Y	E	S	S	N	V	P	N	F
N	D	S	B	X	B	C	V	H	P	N	E	O	R	H	H	J	O	B	X
V	O	E	H	U	J	V	F	U	S	R	F	Z	W	B	F	I	S	A	I
E	O	M	C	M	E	V	W	H	G	V	E	O	V	L	T	V	E	N	E
S	J	E	O	I	C	G	O	A	I	H	O	I	R	A	I	F	O	E	K
T	A	N	F	U	T	Z	L	I	L	O	Y	Q	L	M	N	Y	F	N	B
I	M	T	Q	U	D	A	N	R	B	F	U	S	O	V	A	R	H	E	U
G	E	S	D	P	I	G	X	B	V	T	N	S	K	W	D	T	P	Z	K
A	M	A	X	R	A	T	C	J	H	A	W	Y	H	B	X	R	I	B	A
T	Q	P	T	B	R	R	K	I	R	A	M	C	J	X	J	U	A	O	Z
O	V	G	K	O	I	U	U	T	P	K	E	Y	W	S	H	T	K	D	N
R	T	G	S	Y	E	Y	D	E	N	Z	I	B	R	B	N	U	J	E	A
C	H	A	G	H	S	C	R	B	P	R	O	T	O	C	O	L	M	T	O
V	V	H	Z	R	I	I	N	S	U	R	A	N	C	E	G	U	T	F	L

Investigator CV (Curriculum Vitae), Advertisements, Subject Diaries, Safety Information, ICD (Informed Consent Document), Trial Agreement, IB (Investigator Brochure), ICD (Informed Consent Document) Translations, Protocol, Insurance

Word Search

15. HIPAA (i)

Z	G	Y	V	D	C	A	X	W	N	I	Y	J	O	P	U	L	D	M	Z
U	F	D	D	Z	B	F	C	M	Q	R	C	L	Q	X	H	U	H	M	Z
N	O	W	S	A	V	L	A	X	V	E	J	P	D	F	J	Y	Q	A	G
O	E	C	B	M	C	Q	F	U	F	O	G	H	G	V	S	Q	T	F	M
Y	O	G	O	W	I	R	I	C	T	E	V	E	N	B	S	A	P	J	N
T	G	H	P	V	O	N	G	W	O	H	D	U	E	K	D	T	R	S	P
H	J	A	E	A	E	I	I	U	T	F	O	A	Q	C	T	F	N	R	R
A	J	P	I	A	V	R	S	M	X	G	O	R	I	F	X	J	B	H	E
M	G	L	R	N	L	X	E	J	U	V	D	H	I	R	R	J	Y	K	Z
G	P	X	D	I	N	T	S	D	I	M	P	P	V	Z	I	P	P	J	Z
Q	D	S	B	B	V	S	H	L	E	A	S	N	T	Y	A	P	N	Y	J
Q	F	W	U	H	E	A	L	P	R	N	N	T	G	N	O	T	X	X	G
T	E	Z	Y	R	U	L	C	G	L	X	T	X	A	P	H	I	I	B	U
V	I	I	D	F	P	F	O	Y	L	A	X	I	G	N	B	V	J	O	U
C	H	D	V	J	H	M	Q	T	R	T	N	O	T	T	D	M	C	J	N
F	A	P	B	E	E	L	U	Z	I	U	C	S	K	I	O	A	V	K	W
E	L	H	E	D	K	I	T	S	M	S	L	K	C	W	E	L	R	H	Z
L	G	D	B	T	J	N	A	M	E	S	T	E	S	N	D	S	E	D	E
P	E	Z	I	T	Y	V	B	A	F	Q	N	O	M	W	R	O	H	S	S
J	N	C	L	E	A	R	I	N	G	H	O	U	S	E	S	R	L	K	Y

Address, Demographic Data, PHI (Protected Health Information), Names, Clearing Houses, Authorization, Minimum Standards, Covered Entities, Health Plans, Privacy Rule

Word Search

16. HIPAA (ii)

F	K	C	F	Y	P	C	I	Q	K	B	J	I	U	H	R	Q	D	H	I
L	U	V	I	Z	V	Z	K	G	T	A	O	H	O	E	O	Y	M	E	T
O	L	L	R	F	X	V	C	B	J	M	Z	A	B	H	R	B	X	A	A
X	Z	E	L	Q	R	B	P	P	Z	V	B	M	W	A	Y	I	O	L	V
W	D	K	R	F	Z	X	F	Z	S	T	U	Y	S	S	T	O	I	T	X
R	Q	K	V	N	A	I	U	F	H	N	H	S	L	K	W	M	X	H	H
R	Q	S	K	J	Q	C	O	M	E	H	E	W	D	W	O	E	L	C	F
P	Y	C	X	Y	X	K	E	N	A	C	G	X	P	X	H	T	G	A	G
O	B	V	F	E	S	Z	O	P	E	H	Z	U	D	W	L	R	D	R	I
R	P	V	C	Z	C	H	M	N	H	P	G	S	U	F	Y	I	T	E	H
T	C	I	K	V	P	B	M	H	B	O	R	C	D	P	J	C	X	P	W
A	C	H	Q	E	U	U	U	H	I	I	T	W	H	P	E	D	V	R	G
B	J	E	L	I	M	O	J	J	A	E	P	O	K	F	A	A	K	O	V
I	X	E	V	I	X	D	T	K	Y	C	G	K	G	L	W	T	P	V	Y
L	T	P	N	H	Q	Y	O	F	S	T	Y	W	C	R	P	A	C	I	U
I	E	I	I	T	P	E	N	A	L	T	I	E	S	Y	A	L	M	D	Z
T	M	V	Y	I	D	T	Z	A	Q	H	Z	T	O	B	H	P	Y	E	G
Y	C	E	L	E	M	E	N	T	S	O	F	D	A	T	E	S	H	R	U
M	F	M	A	F	R	Y	F	E	M	A	I	L	A	D	D	R	E	S	S
S	N	M	P	X	V	D	R	F	A	X	N	U	M	B	E	R	J	L	T

Portability, Full Face Photograph, Telephone Number, Minimum Necessary, Penalties, Elements of Dates, email Address, Fax Number, Biometric Data, Healthcare Provider

Word Search

17. Approaches to Drug Discovery

L	E	M	Q	B	J	U	I	Y	Q	I	Q	V	Q	B	Y	M	Z	B	N
I	M	J	U	D	G	O	E	C	V	E	C	B	G	S	M	S	X	O	P
D	F	E	D	P	H	X	X	L	N	X	B	G	M	M	E	H	I	R	R
M	T	Y	D	M	M	T	R	O	O	F	B	K	U	T	O	T	X	O	E
K	C	V	G	N	E	W	D	R	U	G	M	G	A	T	A	P	U	S	C
O	L	N	L	L	U	J	Z	A	P	X	U	D	X	Z	D	D	G	T	L
Z	I	N	J	R	Y	O	R	Q	W	N	I	O	I	G	R	R	B	X	I
H	N	C	R	F	G	B	J	G	X	D	Q	M	J	N	U	U	Z	V	N
I	I	L	K	V	Y	C	C	H	N	U	I	S	C	K	G	G	M	R	I
T	C	Q	D	V	T	C	E	A	M	T	R	R	S	X	S	C	T	P	C
C	A	D	C	A	L	Z	C	K	P	G	M	S	T	R	E	A	I	Y	A
O	L	Q	U	I	H	D	Z	O	M	M	A	V	X	N	L	N	Y	Y	L
M	T	U	L	M	A	A	D	U	G	O	Y	T	O	H	E	D	A	J	T
P	E	A	E	E	L	A	O	G	W	U	L	D	U	X	C	I	G	G	E
O	S	P	L	P	E	V	U	L	Y	V	G	V	I	N	T	D	C	M	S
U	T	E	V	L	N	O	Y	D	S	A	O	X	E	Z	I	A	Q	K	T
N	I	M	H	T	S	O	K	H	M	O	F	K	P	E	O	T	O	R	I
D	N	K	J	V	V	Y	P	Y	K	G	H	E	V	D	N	E	R	M	N
S	G	U	B	T	A	R	G	E	T	S	E	L	E	C	T	I	O	N	G
M	H	W	F	B	W	C	W	X	T	A	I	Y	K	G	O	T	G	R	Y

Hit Compounds, Clinical Testing, New Drug, HTS (High Throughput Screening), Lead Candidates, Lead Optimization, Target Selection, Drug Selection, Drug Candidate, Pre-clinical Testing

Word Search

18. Clinical Trial Support Service Providers for the Sponsor

S	A	J	N	O	Y	T	A	T	D	R	U	G	D	E	P	O	T	C	C
E	V	E	N	T	M	A	N	A	G	E	R	S	I	X	E	O	T	E	E
L	T	G	Q	T	K	V	K	J	N	O	K	S	M	K	M	Y	C	N	N
I	D	H	A	R	Z	P	S	R	E	W	J	X	T	S	C	P	O	T	T
G	Y	X	I	O	S	A	F	U	J	P	L	L	I	N	E	T	U	R	R
W	B	J	M	R	Z	M	U	J	D	O	Y	Z	E	O	C	W	R	A	A
S	D	W	B	P	D	C	U	L	O	L	N	G	V	I	J	X	I	L	L
W	C	E	H	E	V	P	W	U	A	Y	A	N	R	G	U	T	E	L	D
X	P	Z	M	V	Z	X	A	U	F	N	N	C	R	O	J	R	R	A	I
C	W	C	A	S	C	Y	X	R	O	T	J	V	C	Q	A	E	A	B	A
W	O	A	R	A	W	K	D	I	T	Y	Z	B	I	K	V	B	G	Q	G
L	Z	N	P	Q	T	C	T	U	X	Y	T	S	U	U	Y	H	E	N	N
T	L	P	S	Y	K	A	J	C	U	I	A	B	W	A	L	U	N	Y	O
D	V	G	L	U	L	B	O	F	R	U	L	R	D	Y	V	H	C	K	S
T	M	T	R	S	L	V	S	W	J	O	R	Q	C	J	O	F	Y	K	T
V	R	A	N	Y	X	T	W	B	E	I	O	Q	U	H	G	I	D	K	I
I	W	A	F	Z	W	K	A	V	Q	N	R	V	K	P	I	G	N	B	C
J	R	A	L	V	P	X	V	N	B	U	E	J	B	J	R	V	Z	R	S
T	B	G	P	Y	E	G	H	Y	T	L	K	K	E	F	I	F	A	L	V
O	M	R	T	F	B	A	F	W	N	S	O	I	A	Z	Q	X	Y	L	T

Drug Depot, Event Managers, SMO (Site Management Organization), Translation Agency, Consultants, CRO (Contract Research organization), Third Party Archival, Courier Agency, Central Lab, Central Diagnostics

Word Search

19. Data Management

X	S	H	Y	S	V	H	G	M	K	Q	H	A	H	X	T	O	D	Z	D
M	Z	P	A	J	P	N	R	A	Z	L	G	V	F	B	D	C	O	L	V
Q	U	E	R	Y	R	E	S	O	L	U	T	I	O	N	Y	A	U	P	T
M	Q	U	K	S	R	J	D	S	Q	U	J	L	N	Y	G	C	B	B	U
W	F	J	F	R	B	Q	A	K	U	U	T	G	Q	B	K	F	L	E	D
D	A	X	G	Q	T	R	T	V	C	M	O	A	O	F	E	T	E	O	J
A	U	L	Z	E	D	Z	A	P	E	D	C	Y	M	P	C	G	D	H	W
M	R	I	Z	D	A	M	B	R	J	R	F	N	J	X	L	Q	A	V	A
A	H	C	E	V	D	M	A	W	A	Q	N	W	H	X	I	C	T	D	Y
T	Q	M	Z	L	H	Q	S	H	C	J	O	C	W	W	N	T	A	O	X
K	I	H	G	N	C	Z	E	N	Y	O	E	R	Q	V	I	P	E	H	O
J	Q	A	U	H	C	F	D	A	T	A	L	O	C	K	C	U	N	T	V
J	R	P	W	L	Q	Q	E	G	U	M	O	E	P	V	A	V	T	H	T
L	H	J	I	A	C	U	S	G	W	A	E	W	E	Q	L	Y	R	T	O
Z	H	W	R	T	R	F	I	R	K	I	T	L	B	M	C	D	Y	A	R
L	P	W	K	Q	R	K	G	S	T	T	H	T	X	Y	O	W	V	O	R
G	G	C	B	S	L	C	N	F	C	F	G	T	D	D	D	M	S	P	B
D	V	D	C	E	U	W	C	F	T	R	L	G	I	K	I	F	T	R	X
P	Z	Z	X	R	O	D	W	W	W	F	F	Y	L	D	N	P	K	O	Y
M	A	Y	V	K	X	P	P	O	X	T	R	G	Q	W	G	M	H	D	C

Query Resolution, MedDRA (Medical Dictionary for Regulatory Activities), DBQR (Database Quality Review), DCF (Data Clarification Form), EDC (Electronic Data Capture), Data Lock, Database Design, Clinical Coding, Double Data Entry, DVP (Data Validation Plan)

Word Search

20. Seious Adverse Events

W	Q	I	L	D	Y	W	R	Z	Q	P	D	I	Q	Z	Q	M	T	O	X
X	U	R	K	S	E	T	X	X	T	K	Y	K	K	S	G	O	X	D	K
Q	B	K	P	C	U	C	A	N	I	L	S	P	N	P	C	F	Q	Y	D
F	L	C	X	G	E	B	H	O	U	H	E	S	F	E	P	L	I	Y	X
M	O	I	B	P	R	A	J	A	T	T	V	Y	G	M	C	V	L	M	G
T	A	V	F	D	Y	X	J	A	L	D	G	N	D	O	O	A	Z	W	H
I	L	X	E	E	L	E	E	Z	K	L	E	G	A	I	M	L	G	S	O
E	D	V	F	W	T	D	P	E	L	L	E	H	I	O	P	R	N	V	S
Q	I	U	C	A	K	H	X	S	L	Q	Q	N	N	E	L	E	M	Z	P
W	S	N	Z	R	D	S	R	A	A	I	V	A	G	H	I	A	E	Y	I
I	A	Y	Y	S	S	S	H	E	K	E	L	P	N	E	A	S	H	I	T
I	B	Y	K	S	R	C	R	B	A	A	F	Q	X	R	N	T	W	R	A
K	I	W	T	N	E	G	S	V	T	T	B	O	S	V	C	K	T	R	L
W	L	M	T	R	G	K	J	I	O	X	N	M	R	C	E	I	X	K	I
N	I	H	D	U	X	H	N	S	U	O	O	I	U	M	Q	A	D	H	Z
H	T	H	G	C	T	E	W	Q	N	I	M	V	N	C	O	A	R	E	A
O	Y	M	Z	P	G	Q	D	J	C	H	E	G	A	G	M	D	I	G	T
I	R	W	C	N	D	J	A	N	A	A	U	N	V	F	Z	R	K	I	I
W	J	J	O	X	X	B	T	P	I	M	T	R	H	L	S	Y	B	L	O
N	Q	C	K	Z	V	A	W	W	X	W	S	Q	G	V	L	M	W	M	N

Disability, GCP (Good Clinical Practice) Compliance, Hospitalization, De-challenge, SAE (Serious Adverse Event) Form, Life-threatening, Death, Re-challenge, Congenital Anomaly, CIOMS (Council for International Organizations of Medical Sciences)

Word Search

21. Regulatory Authorities

H	A	L	W	Q	D	C	D	G	A	I	B	F	W	Z	T	D	H	Z	Z
G	F	W	H	K	J	X	A	H	P	C	U	W	W	M	J	B	S	I	O
P	B	L	I	W	R	H	R	O	L	B	H	S	R	Z	J	P	Z	D	O
P	L	Z	R	S	T	D	C	G	I	Y	T	P	F	L	I	C	B	D	I
J	X	E	M	V	K	P	T	X	S	O	T	B	D	D	K	R	N	N	N
W	H	U	T	G	I	U	Z	Z	V	C	Q	P	L	J	A	O	Q	K	R
B	A	W	C	M	L	I	S	D	T	D	U	Z	O	Y	I	F	K	A	F
G	F	Q	W	I	H	C	N	Y	Y	A	S	P	K	S	P	R	R	Z	A
D	M	E	C	N	W	O	E	O	O	N	Z	B	S	N	S	I	J	D	U
V	M	T	U	S	I	I	N	O	F	D	O	I	P	Z	T	L	N	X	N
I	D	S	G	P	K	Z	Q	O	G	A	M	U	N	Z	D	N	Y	N	D
E	L	F	Z	E	E	G	H	K	G	R	F	A	K	P	M	H	R	A	Q
D	P	D	A	C	P	K	R	S	E	U	P	G	M	E	A	B	V	J	W
T	E	C	S	T	O	P	Q	P	E	N	T	C	D	X	E	Z	C	Z	R
Y	E	O	D	I	V	J	L	X	E	O	C	A	A	J	V	Q	W	O	N
F	S	S	Y	O	E	A	J	B	M	Z	R	Z	Y	B	Y	K	B	M	M
R	G	N	A	N	I	E	X	C	E	J	J	G	T	U	C	I	Q	F	M
L	X	D	A	R	O	F	V	T	A	N	N	S	P	T	C	N	N	R	E
M	Q	G	T	R	S	S	A	O	X	N	K	G	J	D	C	D	Y	A	O
G	T	L	W	F	M	H	P	O	I	T	J	K	V	S	X	Q	N	X	Z

DCGI (Drugs Controller General of India), US-FDA (Food and Drug Administration), Inspection, ANDA (Abbreviated New Drug Application), EMEA (European Agency for the Evaluation of Medicinal Products), IND (Investigational New Drug), TGA (Therapeutics Goods Administration), Trial Permission, NDA (New Drug Application) MHRA (Medicines and Healthcare Products Regulatory Agency)

Word Search

22. Pharmacovigilance (i)

B	E	I	R	H	H	L	Q	P	E	J	W	Y	Q	Y	I	S	B	Y	J
S	F	N	S	V	E	M	P	R	O	E	R	W	H	G	P	E	A	O	R
K	U	E	W	A	D	Z	C	I	P	L	Q	Q	L	D	R	R	C	C	V
U	H	S	W	L	E	K	M	G	A	U	C	J	L	X	D	I	W	D	C
B	G	M	A	K	A	I	B	F	X	K	R	J	F	O	D	O	X	S	H
O	T	C	D	R	T	C	S	B	D	I	P	M	G	Y	U	U	V	F	G
D	Y	N	X	W	W	A	W	H	W	M	X	Q	F	C	C	S	X	N	U
A	B	U	N	E	X	P	E	C	T	E	D	W	T	G	Y	N	X	K	N
G	H	W	H	R	C	M	V	I	C	B	B	V	K	L	U	E	Z	M	L
O	O	F	A	V	H	D	A	T	V	Y	S	W	F	G	K	S	V	X	I
X	X	L	T	A	D	V	E	R	S	E	E	V	E	N	T	S	I	E	K
V	C	T	V	S	P	C	X	L	Q	U	B	B	D	A	D	R	U	X	E
Q	K	B	O	I	E	O	G	V	D	C	J	F	E	R	S	R	H	D	L
O	R	H	P	I	X	N	Y	G	R	C	O	Q	U	S	Y	N	B	I	Y
G	E	E	R	K	P	J	V	S	J	O	N	C	J	O	T	K	N	H	H
R	N	G	L	Z	E	G	F	S	C	A	U	S	A	L	I	T	Y	S	V
A	N	E	V	A	C	P	A	I	D	X	J	X	B	J	P	T	Z	U	X
H	B	Z	V	S	T	Q	M	G	C	R	Z	A	M	C	X	V	I	R	Z
R	M	V	K	X	E	E	R	V	O	V	W	G	U	Z	U	Z	C	U	G
D	M	B	F	N	D	K	D	F	G	H	N	Z	X	O	J	M	A	S	H

SUSAR (Suspected Unexpected Serious Adverse Reaction), SAE (Serious Adverse Event), Unexpected, Adverse Event, ADR (Adverse Drug Reaction), Seriousness, Unlikely, Causality, Related, Expected

Word Search

23. Pharmacovigilance (ii)

A	X	P	A	R	G	I	Z	J	S	E	P	G	P	D	P	L	A	L	O
R	P	X	M	B	P	J	E	C	W	L	W	O	L	N	X	T	D	Y	H
D	O	D	E	U	V	N	K	M	E	E	U	I	S	J	S	N	S	P	U
F	A	O	L	M	C	I	O	M	S	T	M	L	N	S	Y	Z	U	N	G
Z	J	L	W	S	G	B	W	S	I	B	G	R	Y	L	I	C	W	N	M
K	M	Q	S	E	K	I	X	Y	B	K	U	X	E	D	Q	B	N	N	B
N	Z	V	P	V	B	P	U	M	K	Z	D	T	I	O	U	L	L	B	J
E	F	A	F	E	K	C	J	G	S	G	I	O	Y	J	O	R	V	Y	P
R	K	D	T	R	F	G	H	J	D	N	E	I	L	O	Y	Y	K	R	F
C	Z	Z	U	E	J	R	X	M	I	H	G	B	D	K	L	V	P	O	X
N	G	P	N	X	F	U	C	F	O	F	M	Q	V	B	J	K	J	S	R
S	X	Y	R	Y	V	L	E	M	N	F	J	E	A	Y	W	C	E	A	R
F	D	L	E	K	C	D	Y	W	G	G	E	B	D	D	E	Y	H	L	E
Y	S	Y	L	K	L	P	U	W	Y	F	O	F	W	W	C	E	K	D	R
R	T	S	A	T	A	U	O	O	X	R	G	D	C	D	A	Q	E	Y	A
I	T	V	T	U	D	W	Q	L	P	E	R	V	U	C	D	T	R	T	V
F	U	G	E	S	Y	D	U	Q	D	R	X	A	V	T	F	K	C	A	U
H	A	V	D	P	E	F	E	A	Q	P	L	F	W	H	S	O	X	H	N
I	X	K	T	L	V	M	O	D	E	R	A	T	E	S	P	S	U	R	V
K	J	Z	L	T	Z	S	Y	J	V	W	H	B	N	E	G	K	J	Q	G

CIOMS (Council for International Organizations of Medical Sciences), Severe, Unrelated, Mild, Possibly, Definitely, Probably, Medwatch, Moderate, PSUR (Periodic Safety Update Reports)

Word Search

24. Clinical Trial Documents

T	W	I	E	H	M	E	L	D	V	M	V	L	H	N	D	G	N	G	V
I	P	N	R	M	O	Y	C	Q	J	N	P	F	H	O	F	R	F	T	R
I	R	D	C	E	K	H	J	A	K	R	K	C	T	A	Z	F	I	L	L
Z	V	E	Q	E	Y	P	J	S	V	Y	T	N	X	G	R	Y	A	L	T
P	P	M	P	R	X	O	A	U	U	G	X	I	W	F	I	V	G	F	I
K	G	N	Q	U	J	E	I	T	S	R	X	M	K	W	O	I	P	U	U
Z	X	I	D	C	X	C	I	S	I	U	Z	B	E	R	D	B	R	K	A
P	R	F	K	O	W	C	O	R	L	E	F	Q	P	L	D	N	E	J	K
U	I	I	V	R	M	G	R	S	B	E	N	P	C	F	F	U	F	A	O
C	B	C	H	G	K	T	S	F	Z	A	A	T	M	S	L	S	A	B	I
Y	O	A	W	U	E	V	Z	L	A	Y	P	X	D	O	P	A	I	O	J
F	V	T	F	Y	F	L	W	F	R	B	J	P	C	I	A	R	X	M	N
I	S	I	A	U	T	X	E	O	H	R	P	O	R	N	A	C	N	Q	P
R	P	O	N	W	V	H	T	N	L	B	T	T	T	O	A	R	G	W	Y
I	V	N	G	U	T	A	F	X	S	O	V	W	O	Z	V	X	I	J	N
E	C	A	W	Q	L	V	G	F	R	Y	L	D	E	N	K	A	F	E	F
U	N	D	O	U	G	O	M	P	X	R	S	C	H	M	C	O	L	Z	S
U	X	V	G	Z	V	T	C	I	N	S	U	R	A	N	C	E	K	Z	E
H	E	E	Y	B	H	H	O	O	D	N	D	R	D	V	T	F	P	Y	B
C	R	Y	I	D	M	I	O	Z	Q	D	L	S	G	E	H	S	Q	A	N

Indemnification, ICD (Informed Consent Document), Regulatory Approval, IB (Investigator Brochure), Protocol, CTA (Clinical Trial Agreement), Insurance, Patient Diaries, IRB (Institutional Review Board) Approval, CRF (Case Report Form)

Word Search

25. Source Documents

R	N	U	M	I	C	R	O	F	I	C	H	E	S	F	B	S	K	E	L
E	C	G	F	Y	D	G	Z	Y	E	P	D	K	Y	U	D	D	Z	L	N
C	W	D	Y	Y	W	A	J	C	S	X	P	F	X	R	V	K	M	G	G
L	A	I	B	U	G	E	U	H	O	R	R	G	O	W	E	U	I	G	Z
I	U	P	A	P	O	V	D	U	H	O	W	C	Z	X	R	R	C	G	Z
N	M	E	H	R	T	Y	M	H	P	U	E	T	S	S	T	S	R	M	X
I	F	W	U	Z	X	H	Z	W	F	R	Z	W	L	F	E	B	O	Z	R
C	R	W	U	S	C	O	A	H	Y	Q	R	W	X	I	L	V	F	E	A
A	P	J	I	X	J	O	I	C	V	Q	J	U	R	V	A	O	I	L	Y
L	O	L	T	J	Q	P	A	N	I	Q	J	A	O	R	B	S	L	Y	S
C	O	R	Q	P	L	M	Z	W	W	L	I	D	C	Y	R	V	M	B	G
H	T	M	A	K	R	C	J	M	R	D	B	R	S	R	E	F	S	K	V
A	S	U	V	A	R	C	W	C	T	A	W	N	N	X	P	I	C	O	Y
R	F	U	H	Z	G	E	D	C	R	Q	A	S	K	A	O	B	E	D	M
T	B	P	G	K	N	Y	E	Y	B	C	E	B	J	U	R	U	N	T	O
S	D	G	C	K	M	J	U	J	S	T	U	A	F	G	T	U	K	O	V
M	H	R	U	X	B	K	M	T	D	F	M	C	H	H	S	O	T	Z	L
Q	F	R	Q	U	R	C	C	B	H	D	Z	V	J	Y	K	N	V	Q	E
Y	M	X	S	P	H	O	S	P	I	T	A	L	R	E	C	O	R	D	S
T	O	T	I	K	T	R	R	X	M	G	J	U	O	F	U	A	S	C	N

Microfiches, ECG, Hospital Records, Clinical Charts, Pharmacy Records, Subject Diaries, CT Scans, Lab Reports, Microfilms, X-rays

Word Search

26. Vulnerable Population

O	J	M	X	X	O	F	G	S	A	F	B	U	W	T	N	N	C	D	X
D	I	P	I	N	U	R	S	I	N	G	S	T	U	D	E	N	T	S	P
U	A	Z	X	P	V	G	A	W	P	I	M	T	G	W	S	V	S	A	Q
K	W	W	L	A	G	A	M	P	I	N	G	U	Q	T	M	N	M	R	T
W	E	M	M	G	V	X	V	G	S	D	A	H	N	K	O	R	I	M	X
A	B	X	E	G	W	G	Y	D	A	F	E	E	H	S	J	E	N	E	L
U	U	Y	R	D	U	G	A	O	Z	I	D	Z	R	R	V	U	O	D	U
Z	Z	M	C	E	I	M	R	L	T	U	N	E	R	Z	F	W	R	F	J
A	M	P	B	D	O	C	J	O	T	D	P	D	L	Z	D	Z	I	O	Y
X	K	A	N	N	Y	K	A	S	W	D	F	Y	X	D	S	F	T	R	Q
V	R	L	A	H	E	S	Y	L	E	I	E	F	K	X	D	F	Y	C	K
U	J	C	E	B	E	C	X	Y	S	Y	M	Y	W	Y	K	E	G	E	Q
G	P	V	S	E	A	H	O	D	S	T	R	O	E	V	S	X	R	M	I
V	Z	W	O	M	Y	L	J	H	Z	S	U	E	Q	G	W	R	O	E	Q
H	U	U	R	W	P	B	F	M	L	V	Y	D	F	H	Y	W	U	M	R
X	G	A	Y	M	S	L	I	I	U	N	F	V	E	U	Y	K	P	B	H
I	H	C	E	Z	G	H	P	N	M	A	C	O	V	N	G	V	S	E	C
P	M	N	D	L	L	E	W	O	R	F	X	P	Y	Q	T	E	U	R	T
X	U	H	J	N	C	I	B	R	D	P	W	N	Q	B	X	S	E	S	K
N	J	Z	P	B	K	R	P	S	P	R	I	S	O	N	E	R	S	S	Z

Nursing Students, Nomads, Pharmacy Students, Unemployed Persons, Medical Students, Refugees, Minors, Prisoners, Minority Groups, Armed Force Members

Word Search

27. Investigator Site Evaluation/Qualification

Y	X	X	C	P	A	T	H	U	B	M	B	E	D	D	A	J	K	R	N
Q	S	D	V	N	A	Z	S	X	K	N	H	S	O	D	Y	S	F	O	J
C	C	O	Y	W	I	T	S	M	J	E	S	Y	H	K	C	U	I	J	R
S	S	S	U	C	R	J	I	K	F	E	L	G	O	O	M	T	K	X	E
V	Y	T	O	R	B	F	S	E	I	H	Y	K	Z	A	A	T	J	W	E
K	I	D	U	L	C	Z	V	R	N	B	Y	X	I	C	X	C	G	U	X
G	O	Q	S	D	P	E	O	B	R	T	H	Z	I	M	Y	N	H	D	F
X	T	H	T	B	Y	T	D	O	D	Y	P	F	F	V	A	C	T	P	C
J	R	W	Q	W	A	T	L	O	H	C	I	O	N	X	I	Y	B	H	C
Q	G	Y	F	R	T	V	E	M	C	L	B	B	O	W	Y	I	E	X	E
Z	D	A	O	H	E	W	G	A	A	U	S	B	I	L	R	C	S	A	P
S	K	B	N	Z	W	D	E	U	M	U	M	S	S	Y	O	T	S	G	N
K	A	M	O	B	J	X	Q	K	V	P	X	E	N	D	N	A	U	Y	Z
L	G	S	X	J	J	I	U	H	T	H	H	Z	N	F	E	H	E	S	G
S	F	G	Q	C	P	O	R	H	K	L	K	A	H	T	N	U	S	T	Y
W	O	U	I	R	M	Z	E	H	I	F	Q	X	R	C	S	Q	J	O	T
A	K	E	D	C	T	U	K	H	Q	W	W	M	Z	M	I	Z	V	R	Q
I	N	F	R	A	S	T	R	U	C	T	U	R	E	Q	A	B	X	A	T
P	G	J	Q	Y	O	T	S	D	X	K	S	Y	D	I	O	C	D	G	Q
P	F	A	C	I	L	I	T	Y	V	I	S	I	T	C	E	S	Y	E	E

IRB (Institutional Review Board), Study Team, Source Documents, Pharmacy, Patient Pool, Laboratories, PI Qualification, Storage, Infrastructure, Facility Visit

Word Search

28. Essential Trial Documents (Before the Clinical Phase of the Trial Commences)

L	I	N	S	U	R	A	N	C	E	S	T	A	T	E	M	E	N	T	G
S	A	W	L	M	Y	G	O	Y	E	A	P	V	L	A	J	L	X	T	S
I	D	V	S	U	S	A	K	H	C	I	N	K	M	G	E	I	L	E	Q
G	V	Q	H	O	S	I	U	D	P	U	F	G	K	W	C	A	G	K	I
N	E	I	I	K	E	M	G	V	W	Q	R	S	N	O	V	N	T	X	R
E	R	I	R	C	P	U	Y	N	A	T	U	M	K	O	A	F	M	M	B
D	T	G	B	B	E	V	K	L	E	I	J	J	R	R	Z	F	F	Q	C
A	I	T	A	K	J	B	N	E	K	D	I	P	E	P	T	B	H	M	O
G	S	S	P	Y	Y	Y	S	X	H	U	P	C	X	N	O	Y	O	A	M
R	E	T	P	D	H	H	G	N	I	A	N	R	J	G	J	T	S	Q	P
E	M	D	R	W	V	G	P	Q	Y	E	O	W	O	X	G	W	Q	Q	O
E	E	V	O	Y	B	F	N	R	R	I	Z	T	Y	T	Y	N	E	B	S
M	N	S	V	M	C	F	O	E	P	B	B	X	F	L	O	L	Z	B	I
E	T	B	A	I	K	T	F	U	J	G	F	I	H	R	U	C	L	R	T
N	E	O	L	M	A	E	X	I	I	N	I	Z	F	K	G	W	O	Q	I
T	O	F	B	L	R	M	U	G	Q	E	S	G	M	T	S	Z	A	L	O
S	F	J	U	B	T	H	B	D	R	X	N	X	Q	C	Y	U	N	T	N
Q	W	G	A	O	A	D	R	I	N	A	W	S	D	F	S	Y	B	G	M
V	E	L	Q	F	T	G	U	N	R	B	P	C	E	E	A	E	N	Q	Q
R	Q	W	O	D	P	I	X	U	J	F	I	N	J	L	B	R	K	Q	V

Insurance Statement, Signed Agreements, Advertisement, Signed Protocol, IRB (Institutional Review Board) Approval, IB (Investigator Brochure), ICD (Informed Consent Document), IRB Composition, Regulatory Approval, Lab Reference Ranges

Word Search

29. Essential Trial Documents (During the Clinical Conduct of the Trial)

P	A	C	I	C	O	M	P	L	E	T	E	D	C	R	F	F	V	K	H
R	L	O	P	G	A	B	Z	A	X	X	Q	A	H	U	T	A	R	V	V
O	U	L	A	J	S	J	F	B	C	G	L	O	G	X	W	W	S	X	S
T	V	K	C	D	I	V	P	X	Q	B	H	R	F	T	D	G	O	E	K
O	M	N	C	Q	G	C	M	M	X	C	Q	V	U	K	O	P	U	U	P
C	C	X	O	S	N	M	D	S	X	B	L	X	G	L	K	F	R	E	C
O	M	B	U	P	E	A	Q	A	V	Z	Z	P	T	Z	V	X	C	T	R
L	D	M	N	U	D	W	R	H	M	A	G	N	E	B	Y	K	E	V	Z
A	C	J	T	S	I	V	R	H	I	E	E	X	I	R	F	R	D	C	C
M	I	P	A	E	C	R	I	J	U	M	N	Q	R	S	O	K	O	N	A
E	G	H	B	T	D	N	Y	B	L	W	T	D	F	N	S	V	C	S	E
N	Q	R	I	Z	M	E	N	O	U	U	I	B	M	E	F	U	U	C	R
D	E	W	L	W	H	U	R	F	B	P	N	K	S	E	C	E	M	H	U
M	W	Z	I	Z	K	N	M	K	X	E	D	J	G	Z	N	W	E	O	P
E	F	T	T	Z	E	N	M	U	D	Q	K	A	G	W	Z	T	N	R	N
N	L	E	Y	Y	G	H	E	T	X	K	Q	T	T	Q	J	F	T	G	W
T	X	S	L	X	K	U	G	P	Y	H	B	T	O	E	W	W	S	X	K
D	T	M	O	N	I	T	O	R	I	N	G	R	E	P	O	R	T	S	A
U	F	X	G	P	N	E	H	E	U	J	U	E	B	L	U	Q	F	S	Q
Q	J	W	S	A	S	C	R	E	E	N	I	N	G	L	O	G	O	Q	Z

Protocol Amendment, IP Accountability Logs, Signed ICD (Informed Consent Document), Source Documents, Completed CRF (Case Report Form), Monitoring Reports, Screening Log, IB (Investigator Brochure) Update, ICD (Informed Consent Document) Amendment, Enrolment Log

Word Search

30. Essential Trial Documents (After Completion or Termination of the Trial)

S	U	B	J	E	C	T	I	D	C	O	D	E	L	I	S	T	E	Z	E
F	I	N	A	L	P	A	Y	M	E	N	T	R	E	C	O	R	D	G	I
V	I	P	A	C	C	O	U	N	T	A	B	I	L	I	T	Y	N	S	A
Y	N	M	I	A	R	C	H	I	V	E	L	O	C	A	T	I	O	N	U
V	D	P	J	P	J	T	H	X	H	G	D	B	B	S	T	M	X	W	D
F	P	Z	Z	A	D	Y	X	A	X	A	D	K	S	R	A	B	D	F	I
N	Y	G	S	G	Y	E	Q	B	W	D	T	V	O	C	S	S	P	I	T
W	I	M	N	J	U	V	S	H	I	B	D	P	N	Y	Z	D	B	T	C
W	C	C	R	J	G	U	U	T	D	L	E	C	P	W	F	S	V	S	E
I	N	E	F	L	N	E	T	F	R	R	N	I	S	H	Z	R	U	F	R
X	X	U	O	I	J	K	C	N	Y	U	V	J	P	F	Y	E	M	A	T
W	A	Q	R	Q	C	T	H	R	M	C	C	S	S	L	D	V	Y	S	I
V	S	I	T	E	C	L	O	S	E	O	U	T	R	E	P	O	R	T	F
P	X	B	C	W	A	T	U	R	U	S	R	Y	I	F	L	V	I	Q	I
V	J	N	S	F	A	C	Z	C	W	M	Z	I	R	O	S	R	Y	I	C
T	L	C	Y	L	J	H	B	F	V	M	U	H	F	W	N	H	Q	P	A
U	M	W	U	B	O	S	I	G	N	E	D	C	S	R	Z	L	W	E	T
G	Z	G	W	A	U	K	E	R	I	P	M	U	G	K	K	U	O	I	E
G	E	R	F	Q	B	G	U	T	R	I	B	J	L	U	B	C	J	G	T
R	D	R	M	G	B	Z	I	R	B	R	E	P	O	R	T	I	N	G	S

Subject ID Code List, Final Payment Record, IP Accountability, Archive Location, Site Close-out Report, Signed CSR, IRB Reporting, IP Destruction Logs, Regulatory Reporting, Audit Certificate

Word Search

31. Clinical Trial Terminologies

B	C	C	B	Y	J	A	E	U	I	K	H	S	O	Y	P	Y	I	C	N
O	L	Y	Y	K	W	S	D	V	W	R	D	V	A	O	I	F	N	A	P
K	I	I	Y	P	M	L	T	R	C	A	N	W	Q	G	V	O	S	X	D
U	S	T	N	Q	X	Z	H	P	A	N	O	N	Y	Y	G	X	P	F	F
R	I	R	N	D	Z	A	Z	D	R	D	V	V	N	Z	Y	K	E	N	G
T	K	R	P	U	I	H	H	D	E	O	J	X	R	B	T	G	C	S	E
R	R	O	R	O	C	N	B	E	P	M	R	J	Z	V	W	C	T	X	R
I	S	C	Y	X	W	H	G	F	O	I	R	D	I	T	Z	C	I	Y	I
A	P	J	B	K	K	B	Q	J	E	Z	U	V	W	S	R	G	O	L	X
L	C	S	S	R	K	M	S	Z	Z	A	U	C	H	Y	H	U	N	D	C
S	B	N	C	H	Y	P	Z	N	N	T	H	O	Z	A	J	F	V	J	X
I	O	U	Y	F	K	R	T	N	O	I	J	M	J	T	U	J	P	K	C
T	U	S	H	Y	O	O	E	X	K	O	N	P	K	V	V	Z	J	N	K
E	W	I	B	L	O	K	A	G	A	N	A	L	P	P	C	S	L	G	T
G	D	S	N	S	J	P	C	W	F	L	Z	I	Z	T	R	U	A	C	L
G	S	O	U	R	C	E	D	A	T	A	X	A	N	T	O	R	Y	E	N
R	G	H	G	O	Z	F	C	I	J	U	E	N	K	P	Y	S	S	I	T
O	A	O	V	W	O	X	V	M	M	R	O	C	Y	O	N	F	G	J	L
H	Q	G	E	C	X	C	Y	X	S	R	X	E	K	Y	L	J	W	X	V
L	Z	Q	W	A	U	D	I	T	T	R	A	I	L	B	G	E	E	X	M

Trial Site, Randomization, Compliance, Inspection, Blinding, ADR (Adverse Drug Reaction), SOP (Standard Operating Procedure), SAE (Serious Adverse Event), Source Data, Audit Trail

4

Keys for Odd-One-Out

This section contains solution of 15 exercises pertaining to a particular clinical trial element/activity/process.

Odd-One-Out

1. Marketing Authorization
2. Drug Launch
3. Translation of Informed Consent Document
4. Nurse
5. Safety Reporting to Regulatory Authorities
6. Safety Reporting to Ethics Committee
7. Procurement of Import/Export License
8. Case Report Form Completion
9. Non Confidentiality
10. Adverse Event of Severe Nature
11. Data Validation Plan
12. Review of Signed ICF
13. Drug Launch
14. MEDWATCH
15. Review of Interim Analysis Data to Advise the Study Sponsors whether to Continue or Terminate the Trial

5

Keys for Process Flows

This section contains solution of 20 exercises based on clinical research processes.

Process Flows

1. - Lead Candidates
   - New Drug
2. - Regulatory Submission of IND
   - New Drug Application (NDA)
3. - Protocol
   - Investigator Brochure (IB)
   - Informed Consent Document (ICD)
   - Handling and Storage
   - Collection of Analytical Data
4. - Investigator's Training Meeting
   - Last Patient Visit (LPV)
   - Trial Closure
5. - Obtain information on the Composition, Charter and Functioning of the ERB
   - Visit the facility including Lab, Pharmacy, Wards, ICU, Medical record section, Research room (if any) and Radiological facility etc. in order to ascertain the compliance with the protocol, GCP and applicable regulatory guidelines
   - Forward Essential Documents for EC Submission
6. - Preparation of Minutes of the Meeting to address the queries that remains unanswered along with other issues
   - Circulating the Minutes of the Meeting to all the participating sites for reading before initiating the trial
7. - Preparation of Site Initiation Visit (SIV) report for management review and sign-off
   - Forwarding the SIV report to the site re-iterating the issues and actionable
8. - Clinical Trial Monitoring
9. - Subject reads the ICD in Vernacular Language
   - Investigator/Designee signs the ICD in the presence of Subject
10. - Verbal Consent is obtained from the Subject
    - Subject's Legally Acceptable Representative (LAR) signs and dates the ICD in the presence of Subject and Investigator/Designee
11. - Subject or Subject's Legally Acceptable Representative ask the queries (if any) to the Investigator/Designee
    - Subject receives a copy of signed ICD
12. - Translation of ICD in Vernacular Language(s) by the Agency
    - Translation Approval by Designated Personnel

Process Flows

13. - Site reports the SAE to the Sponsor (within 24 hours) in the prescribed format
    - Site reports all SAEs and follow-up information to the respective EC/IRB/IEC
14. - Sponsor's Designee Receives the SAE and Document the date and time of receipt
    - Sponsor's Designee Reports SAEs to the Applicable Regulatory Authority as per the stipulated timeframe
15. - Investigational Product(s) Storage and Accountability
    - GCP and Applicable Regulatory Guidelines
    - Documentation of Deviations and Actionable
16. - Impact of Deviation on the conduct of study
    - Action Plan and Responsibility
    - Sharing of information with other sites and reporting to EC/IEC/IRB
17. - Data Entry
    - Data Lock
18. - Review of Master Drug Accountability logs for 100% reconciliation
    - Review of final report to EC/IEC/IRB
    - Discussion with Investigator on Regulatory Audits/Inspection as well as Clinical Study Report process and Publication Policies
19. - Preparation of Clinical Study Report
    - Study Close-out
20. - NAI (No Action Indicated)
    - VAI (Voluntary Action Indicated)
    - OAI (Official Action Indicated: probation, civil proceedings, criminal proceedings, consent agreement, disqualification)

Made in United States
North Haven, CT
04 November 2026

21728894R10117